AJPH
A PUBLICATION OF THE
AMERICAN PUBLIC HEALTH ASSOCIATION

AMERICAN JOURNAL of PUBLIC HEALTH
JANUARY 2023
Issue 1

A DIGITAL JOURNAL FOR A GREENER EARTH

AJPH in 2023: Embracing Digital First, p. 5

EMERGING METHODS IN PUBLIC HEALTH

Methods & Population Health Push–Pull Relationship, p. 35
Small Area Estimation, p. 40
Sequential Multiple Assignment Randomized Trial,
pp. 37 and 49
Microrandomized Trials, p. 60

Also in this issue:

UNDERGRADUATE PUBLIC HEALTH
Degree Trends, 2001–2020,
pp. 9 and 115

COMMUNITY-BASED
PARTICIPATORY RESEARCH
Synergy With Antiracism, p. 70

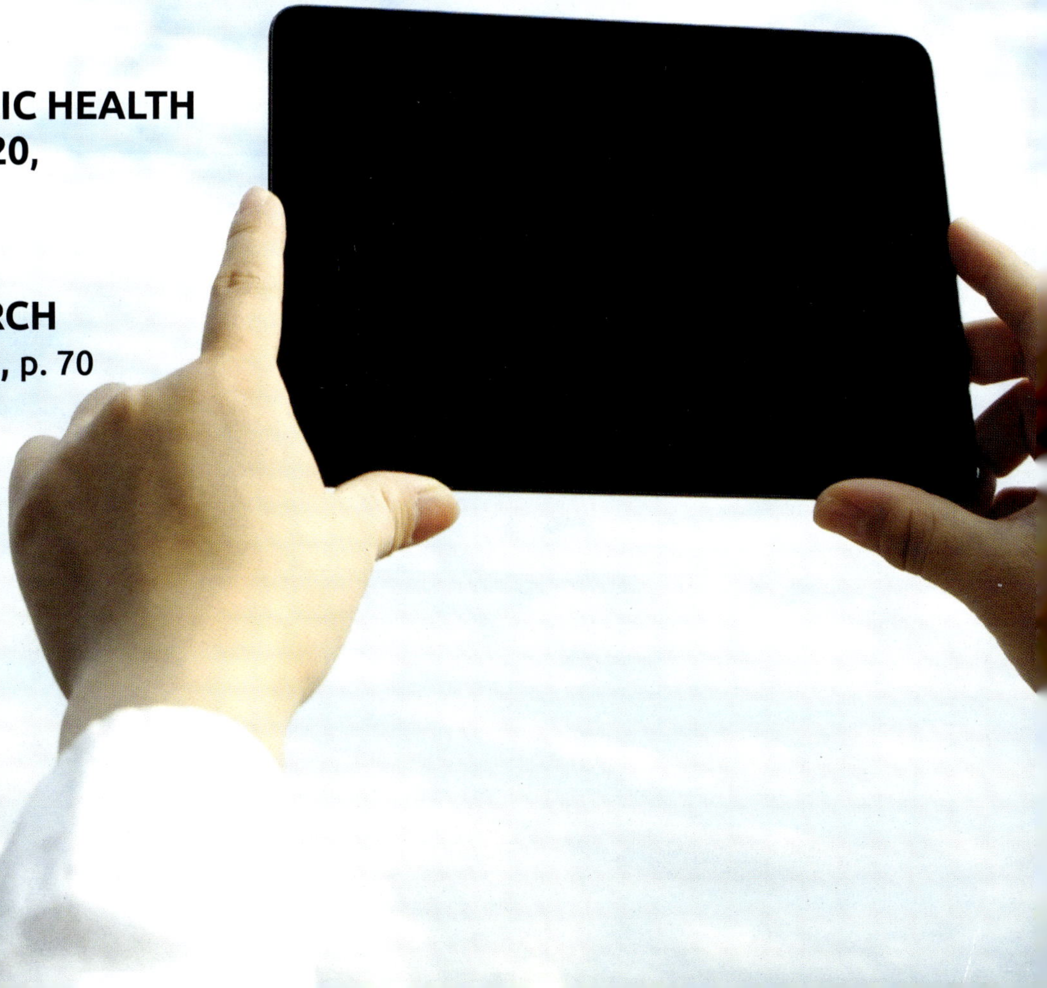

APHA
AMERICAN PUBLIC HEALTH ASSOCIATION
For science. For action. For health.

AJPH®, published monthly, is the official Journal of the American Public Health Association®, 800 I St NW, Washington, DC 20001-3710; (202) 777- APHA; TDD (202) 777-2500. APHA is a nongovernmental professional society founded in 1872, representing all disciplines and specialties in public health.

The *American Journal of Public Health*® (*AJPH*) (print ISSN: 0090-0036; electronic ISSN: 1541- 0048), first published in 1911, is the official journal of the American Public Health Association® (APHA). The oldest and largest organization of public health professionals in the world, APHA represents approximately 30 000 members from more than 50 occupations of public health.

Submissions: Visit www.editorialmanager.com/ajph or ajph.edmgr.com for online manuscript preparation and submission guidelines. Contributions of original unpublished research, social science analyses, scholarly essays, critical commentaries, departments, and letters to the editor are welcome. Questions? Write ajph.submissions@apha.org or call APHA at (202) 777-2469.

Print plus online subscriptions: Institutional price (print copy with online access for a single institution and all authorized users, regardless of geographic location) varies by size of organization and ranges from $993–$1445 for US organizations, and $1073–$1526 for international organizations (air delivery); multiple campuses not permitted without special arrangement. Details of the tiered pricing system at https://subscriptionoffice.com/pages/apha-landing-page. To order, write apha.subscriptions@apha.org.

Online only subscriptions: Institutional price for one institution and its authorized users (regardless of geographic location) is $878–$1307. To order, write apha.subscriptions@apha.org. For academic consortia or multisite corporate subscriptions, contact apha.subscriptions@apha.org.

Print-only subscriptions: Institutional price is US $701, $782 international.

Back print issues: A limited number of print issues are for sale. Single copies are US $49, $55 international (air delivery). Shipping included; prepay only. To order, write apha.subscriptions@apha.org.

Reprints: For prices and ordering information on 50 or more reprints, check the Reprints section at www.ajph.org. To order smaller quantities of reprints (rush delivery), use the "Purchase Article" link on the article site itself.

Electronic access: Online articles more than 10 years old are available free for personal use at www.ajph.org. Recent articles are available through pay-per-view: single PDF article for $24, single issue access for 24 hours for $33, or entire site access for 24 hours for $38.

Postal information: Periodicals postage paid at Washington, DC, and additional mailing offices. Postmaster: Send address changes to American Journal of Public Health, 800 I St NW, Washington, DC 20001-3710.

Address changes: Send to AJPH, Membership Department (members) or AJPH Subscriptions (subscribers), APHA, 800 I St NW, Washington, DC 20001-3710. Or write to membership.mail@apha. org (members) or apha.subscriptions@apha.org (subscribers).

Advertising: For pricing and other information, see www.ajph.org. Please write to ashell.alston@apha.org or call (202) 777-2470 for other advertising opportunities. Ask about special exhibit packages and sponsorships. Acceptance of advertising by the *Journal* does not imply endorsement of products.

Indexes: Publications that index or abstract articles from AJPH include the following: Ageline, Assia (Applied Social Science Index and Abstracts), Biological Abstracts, Chemical Abstracts, CINAHL, Criminal Justice Abstracts, EMBASE, EMCare, Environmental Abstracts, e-psyche, ERIC, ETOH (Alcohol and Alcohol Problems Science Database), Excerpta Medica, Food Science and Technology, General Science Index, Grateful Med, Hospital Literature Index, Human Resources Abstracts, International Pharmaceutical Abstracts (IPA), Medline, Physical Education Index, Pollution Abstracts, Psychological Abstracts, PsychINFO, Safety Science Abstracts, Sage Family Studies Abstracts, Sage Human Resources Abstracts, Science Citation Index, SCOPUS, SIIC Data Bases, Social Work Research and Abstracts, and Statistical Reference Index (SRI)/LexisNexis.

AJPH

A PUBLICATION OF THE
AMERICAN PUBLIC HEALTH ASSOCIATION

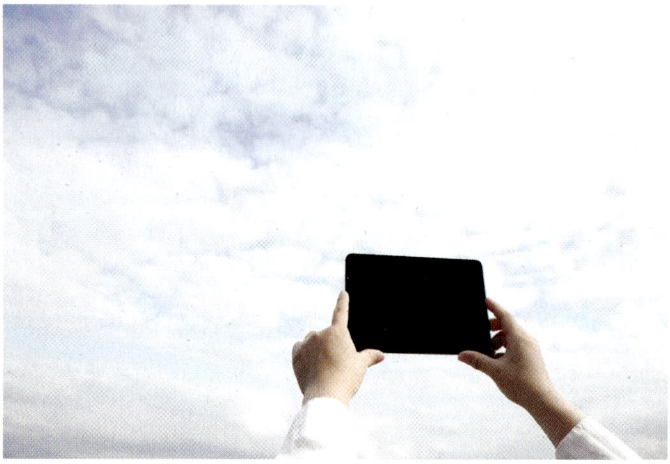

COVER: A change has been brewing in how people want information and how associations and other publishers provide content. We are delighted to announce that *AJPH* is embracing this shift. During 2023 we will be transitioning *AJPH* to a digital-first publication. Many positive impacts come with this change: reduced printing, expanded digital offerings, reallocated resources such as short video, podcasts, and more. We hope you're as excited about the coming changes as we are.

Cover concept and selection by Aleisha Kropf. Photo by Kohei Hara, courtesy of Getty Images. Printed with permission.

APHA
AMERICAN PUBLIC HEALTH ASSOCIATION
For science. For action. For health.

Promoting public health research, policy, practice, and education is the *AJPH* mission. As we widen our scope to embrace global issues, we also sharpen our focus to support the needs of public health practitioners. We invite contributions of original unpublished research, opinion and commentary, and letters to the editor.

The *Journal* is printed on acid-free recycled paper.

OPEN ACCESS · ONLINE ONLY · PODCAST · DATA SUPPLEMENT AVAILABLE

EDITOR'S CHOICE

5 *AJPH* in 2023: Embracing Digital-First
G. C. Benjamin

OPINIONS, IDEAS, & PRACTICE

EDITORIALS

6 Wastewater Surveillance—“Messy” Science With Public Health Potential
J. W. Keck and S. M. Berry

9 Two Decades of Progress in Undergraduate Public Health: Where Do We Go From Here?
R. K. Riegelman

12 Environmental Justice From Pennsylvania to Paris: A Public Health of Consequence, January 2023
F. Kapadia

PERSPECTIVES

15 Extreme Heat Governance: A Critical Analysis of Heat Action Plans in California
M. T. Schmeltz, J. A. Smith, I. Olmos, and E. Quintero

20 Rethinking “Herd” Mentalities and Rethinking the Value of the History of Public Health
J. Steere-Williams

22 Pornography Use and Public Health: Examining the Importance of Online Sexual Behavior in the Health Sciences
J. B. Grubbs, C. G. Floyd, and S. W. Kraus

27 Cigarette Use Among Older Adults: A Forgotten Population
B. A. Kleykamp and J. A. Kulak

NOTES FROM THE FIELD

30 Social Disparities in the Duration of Power and Piped Water Outages in Texas After Winter Storm Uri
S. E. Grineski, T. W. Collins, J. Chakraborty, E. Goodwin, J. Aun, and K. D. Ramos

EMERGING METHODS IN PUBLIC HEALTH

35 Embracing Advanced Methodology to Improve Population Health
R. Vaughan

37 Adaptive Interventions for a Dynamic and Responsive Public Health Approach
N. J. Seewald

RESEARCH & ANALYSIS

EMERGING METHODS IN PUBLIC HEALTH

40 A Novel Bayesian Spatial–Temporal Approach to Quantify SARS-CoV-2 Testing Disparities for Small Area Estimation
C. Bauer, X. Li, K. Zhang, M. Lee, E. Guajardo, S. Fisher-Hoch, J. McCormick, M. E. Fernandez, and B. Reininger

49 The Sequential Multiple Assignment Randomized Trial for Controlling Infectious Diseases: A Review of Recent Developments
X. Wang and B. Chakraborty

60 Microrandomized Trials: Developing Just-in-Time Adaptive Interventions for Better Public Health
X. Liu, N. Deliu, and B. Chakraborty

PERSPECTIVES FROM THE SOCIAL SCIENCES

70 Antiracism and Community-Based Participatory Research: Synergies, Challenges, and Opportunities
P. J. Fleming, L. C. Stone, M. S. Creary, E. Greene-Moton, B. A. Israel, K. D. Key, A. G. Reyes, N. Wallerstein, and A. J. Schulz

SURVEILLANCE

79 Timing and Trends for Municipal Wastewater, Lab-Confirmed Case, and Syndromic Case Surveillance of COVID-19 in Raleigh, North Carolina
N. Kotlarz, D. A. Holcomb, A. B. M. Tanvir Pasha, S. Reckling, J. Kays, Y.-C. Lai, S. Daly, S. Palani, E. Bailey, V. T. Guidry, A. Christensen, S. Berkowitz, J. A. Hoppin, H. Mitasova, L. S. Engel, F. L. de los Reyes, and A. Harris

OPEN-THEMED RESEARCH

89 Effect of the COVID-19 Global Pandemic on Illinois Children Tested for Blood Lead Level and Exposure
F. D. Fokum, T. Entezar, and K. McAfee

96 SARS-CoV-2 Infection, Hospitalization, and Death in Vaccinated and Infected Individuals by Age Groups in Indiana, 2021–2022
W. Tu, P. Zhang, A. Roberts, K. S. Allen, J. Williams, P. Embi, and S. Grannis

105 A Community Health Worker–Based Intervention on Anthropometric Outcomes of Children Aged 3 to 21 Months in Urban Pakistan, 2019–2021
A. S. Shonchoy, A. A. Akram, M. Khan, H. Khalid, S. Mazhar, A. Khan, and T. Kurosaki

115 Trends in Degree Conferrals, Degree-Associated Debt, and Employment Outcomes Among Undergraduate Public Health Degree Graduates, 2001–2020
J. P. Leider, E. Burke, R. H. N. Nguyen, C. Plepys, C. Kirkland, B. Resnick, and L. Magaña

BACKMATTER

OTHER DEPARTMENTS

128 Subscription Form

ERRATUM

e1 Erratum In: “The Opioid Industry Documents Archive: A Living Digital Repository”

AJPH in 2023: Embracing Digital-First

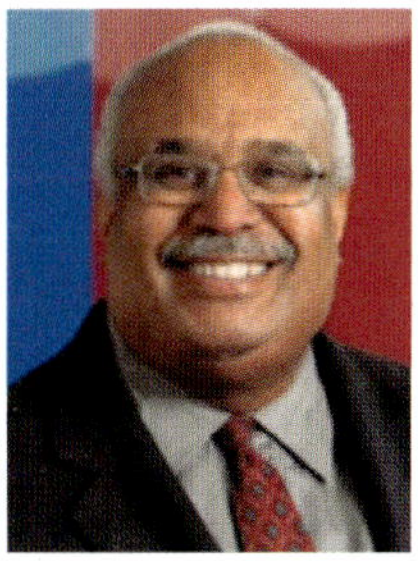

Over the past few decades, a change has been brewing in how people want information and how associations and other publishers provide content. The Web and digital versions of newspapers, for example, have become increasingly important as readers have shifted away from having physical papers delivered to their homes. People want and expect instant access to information.

We've watched these changes for years and taken action to meet them and the changing desires of our members and *AJPH* subscribers. *AJPH* articles have been available online for years. We've released First Look articles as a way to share information more quickly. Fifteen years ago, we even moved the *AJPH* version of record from our print edition to the digital one.

Over the past three years, as the world dealt with COVID-19, the shift to digital really ramped up within the publishing and news industries, especially for associations.

Looking at trends within the industry and our membership, member comments, and what we offer, we've decided to embrace this shift and spend 2023 transitioning *AJPH* to a digital-first publication. I'll miss flipping through the glossy pages of *AJPH*, but it's time to readjust our thinking and continue the evolution of *AJPH* to ensure that it maintains its status as the leading resource for impactful public health research and information.

The positive impacts are many: *AJPH* will reduce its contribution to the climate crisis by reducing the number of copies of the journal being printed and mailed, our digital offerings will expand, and resources will be reallocated to more popular and effective mediums, including short videos, podcasts, and more.

We hope you're as excited about the coming changes as we are.

Of course, this was not an easy decision. Providing print copies of the journal to members who want them is an APHA member benefit, and we don't want to change the format of that benefit unless the positives vastly outweigh the negatives. In this instance, we believe that's the case.

To show our ongoing commitment to members and readers who desire it, we're developing a full-issue PDF to provide a cover-to-cover experience for those who wish to receive it as part of their APHA membership. People will be able to print the PDF and save it to up to six devices. We're making upgrades to the *AJPH* e-Reader edition as well, which will be available as an individual purchase with a discount for members or at a reduced monthly subscription rate.

For members accustomed to receiving *AJPH* in print, the shift will happen at your renewal date. As you renew, you'll have an opportunity to receive the new full-issue PDF. Of course, all members will continue to enjoy full access to all *AJPH* articles, including those dating back to 1911.

Print is not disappearing entirely, it's simply not at the forefront anymore. Organizations subscribing to *AJPH* outside of any APHA membership will be able to purchase *AJPH* in print to make it available as a resource in their libraries if they wish. In instances where someone wants to purchase a physical issue, we'll print the needed copies on-demand.

We hope you'll join us in embracing these changes in the same spirit that we made them, with an eye toward a more versatile, accessible, and climate-friendly *AJPH*. For more information on this transition, check out our FAQs at www.apha.org/ajph and stay tuned to the journal's home page, www.ajph.org, for updates. AJPH

Georges C. Benjamin, MD
Executive Director
American Public Health Association

DOI: https://doi.org/10.2105/AJPH.2022.307161

19 Years Ago

Pitfalls of and Controversies in Cluster Randomization Trials

The issue of choosing the unit of inference is sometimes referred to as the "unit of analysis problem." We believe that this phrase can be misleading, since it confuses the choice of analytic unit with the need to account for clustering. Similarly, statements sometimes seen in the literature to the effect that "analysis by individual" is incorrect for cluster randomization trials or that the "allocation unit should be the unit of analysis" are also misleading. In general, an analysis at the individual level that properly accounts for the effect of clustering is equivalent to an appropriately weighted cluster-level analysis. Thus, the issue of fundamental importance in this context is best referred to as the unit of inference, rather than the unit of analysis.

From AJPH, March 2004, p. 418

47 Years Ago

A Bayesian Approach To Health Project Estimation

[A]nyone trying to study anything in a poor country hears time and again that practically any statistic he finds is useless. Admitting this, he must decide what to do next. There are three possible approaches. The first rejects statistical analysis and depends on the opinion of individuals with long experience in the field. . . . The second approach ignores the problem and proceeds to apply the whole gamut of classical statistical methods to the existing data. . . . There is a third way . . . Bayesian statistical techniques can create a measure of output in a way that lays all the assumptions open to refutation, but also permits the use of expert opinion where recorded numbers are nonexistent or hopelessly inadequate.

From AJPH, August 1976, p. 748

Wastewater Surveillance—"Messy" Science With Public Health Potential

James W. Keck, MD, MPH, and Scott M. Berry, PhD, MBA

ABOUT THE AUTHORS

James W. Keck is with the Department of Family and Community Medicine, College of Medicine, University of Kentucky, Lexington. Scott M. Berry is with the Department of Mechanical Engineering, College of Engineering, University of Kentucky.

See also Kotlarz et al., p. 79.

Wastewater testing for infectious diseases blossomed during the COVID-19 pandemic.[1] Public health agencies are using wastewater data to augment traditional case and syndromic disease surveillance systems.[2] In this issue of *AJPH*, Kotlarz et al. (p. 79) report on the correspondence between COVID-19 disease trends observed with wastewater analysis, clinical testing, and syndromic surveillance in Raleigh, North Carolina, in 2020. They found moderate to strong correlations in COVID-19 trends across these data sources with wastewater influent and clinical testing disease signals preceding disease signals from syndromic surveillance and wastewater solids.

Wastewater analysis is an emerging surveillance tool that has potential benefits but also presents challenges compared with existing disease surveillance approaches. We find it useful to think about wastewater surveillance in the paradigm of a SWOT (strengths, weaknesses, opportunities, and threats) analysis (Figure 1). Kotlarz et al. identified some of these issues as pros and cons in the first figure in their article.

Wastewater analysis as a disease surveillance tool has several potential advantages over traditional surveillance methods. Wastewater analysis theoretically provides information about all of the individuals contributing to the wastewater—in essence, pooled testing of a community. Kotlarz et al. measured disease biomarkers in wastewater samples that may have contained contributions from more than 500 000 individuals living in Raleigh. Compared with individual clinical testing, wastewater analysis is efficient and likely cost saving—one study estimated that it was 1.7% of the total cost of clinical testing.[3]

Unlike syndromic and case-based disease surveillance, wastewater analysis does not rely on an individual having access to or seeking health care. As the title to the popular children's book by Taro Gomi proclaims, *Everyone Poops*. For this reason, wastewater surveillance can increase health equity if deployed in populations with less access to clinical testing or health care. Marginalized, rural, and resource-poor communities and their associated public health institutions stand to benefit from timely wastewater disease data that can inform local decision-making and the community members. As more individuals turn to home-based rapid tests and as the frequency of mild or asymptomatic COVID-19 cases increases, syndromic and case-based disease surveillance may further underestimate disease prevalence. In these situations, wastewater analysis will still identify trends in community disease burden, such as during the recent Omicron variant–fueled waves of COVID-19 infections.[4]

Although wastewater surveillance is an excellent complement to traditional disease surveillance, it has limitations. Wastewater samples positive for severe acute respiratory syndrome coronavirus 2 (SARS-CoV-2) viral RNA cannot tell us who in the community is infected. However, there are many reports of wastewater surveillance triggering enhanced clinical testing to identify infected individuals, such as happened in Yellowknife, Canada.[5] Kotlarz et al. also recognize that wastewater analysis cannot distinguish between individuals with new and those with convalescing infections. Nor do we know with confidence who is contributing to a community's wastewater. Populations are dynamic, and individuals have varied toileting behaviors. Some individuals residing in a community will leave for work or recreation, and visitors from outside the community will make "deposits" into the wastewater system. There is also substantial variation in the amount of virus an infected individual deposits into the system—not all infected individuals shed virus in their feces, viral shedding may last from days to weeks, and shedding intensity varies over many magnitudes[6]—likely because of a combination of host (e.g., age, illness severity, prior immunity) and virus (e.g., variant, infective dose) characteristics.

The tidal wave of enthusiasm for wastewater surveillance in the research and public health communities presents

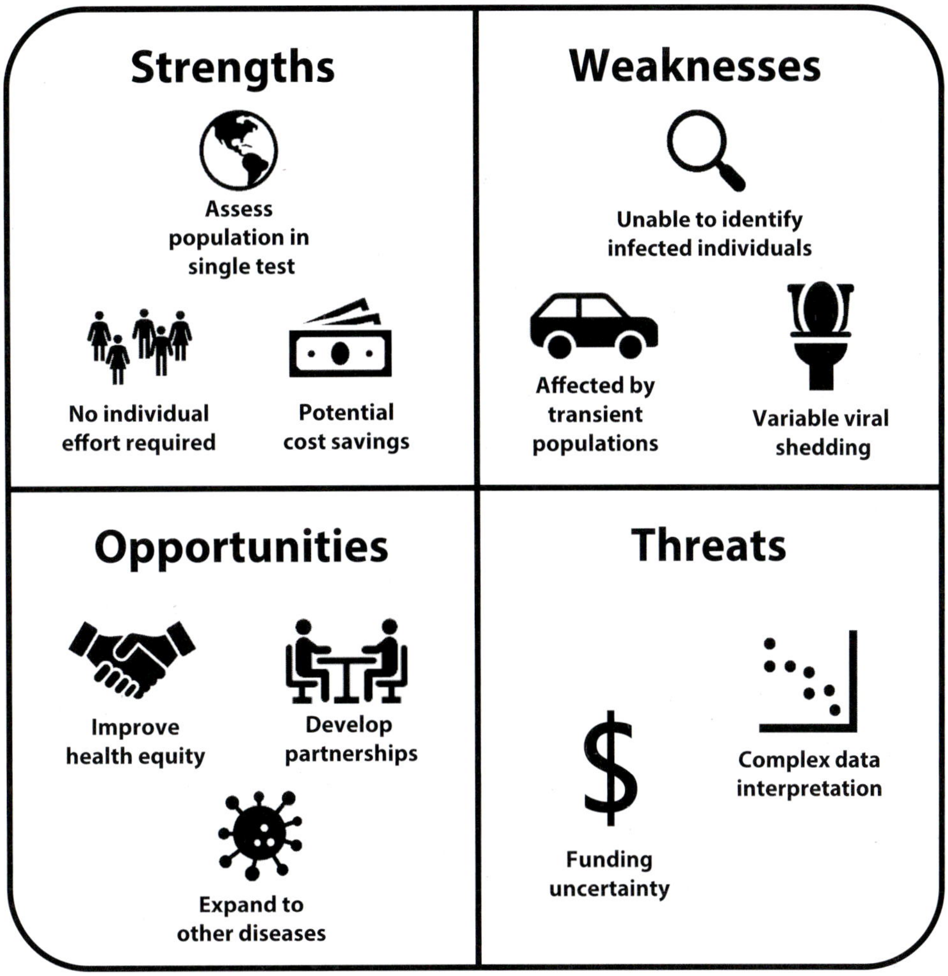

FIGURE 1— **Strengths, Weaknesses, Opportunities, and Threats (SWOT) Analysis of Wastewater Testing as a Public Health Disease Surveillance Tool**

an opportunity to build on the successes of this approach. As exemplified by the Raleigh wastewater study authors' affiliations, implementing wastewater surveillance fosters multidisciplinary and multiorganizational collaborations. Scientists, public utilities operators, engineers, epidemiologists, and others worked together to conduct the wastewater study. Partnerships like these are critical for addressing complex public health problems.

Wastewater analysis can and should look beyond estimates of COVID-19 disease trends. Wastewater surveillance detected a subclinical outbreak of polio in Israel in 2013 and informed targeted vaccine campaigns.[7] Less than a decade later, wastewater surveillance in New York State helped define the spread of a vaccine-derived poliovirus outbreak following its detection in a hospitalized patient.[8] The wastewater partnerships and infrastructure developed during the COVID-19 pandemic likely made the rapid pivot to wastewater testing for polio possible and can enable other critical disease (e.g., monkeypox) surveillance activities.

Community circulation of SARS-CoV-2 and poliovirus are only the beginning of what we can learn from wastewater analysis. With advances in molecular biology and genetic sequencing, laboratories are sequencing wastewater to track SARS-CoV-2 variants,[9] measuring levels of antimicrobial resistance genes,[10] and looking for novel viruses that could cause the next pandemic. The utility of wastewater analysis goes beyond infectious disease surveillance: scientists are testing wastewater for many biomarkers of public health importance, such as pharmaceutical metabolites[11] and markers of exposure to air pollution.[12]

Wastewater surveillance is a particularly attractive public health tool for communities with limited access to clinical testing or health care. However, these same communities may also lack laboratory infrastructure, human resources, and external partnerships as well as centralized sanitation systems. Hence, there is an opportunity for community-engaged research to design wastewater analysis approaches that meet the needs of these communities. Strategies that build local capacity, emphasize simplified analytic tests, and cultivate partnerships between local stakeholders can maximize the potential of wastewater disease surveillance across a diversity of settings.

Wastewater analysis as a disease surveillance modality faces potential threats. As with other public health programs, the availability of resources (i.e., funding) will influence the sustainability of wastewater surveillance initiatives. The Centers for Disease Control and Prevention has provided laboratory capacity grants to many states to enhance their wastewater surveillance programs. Wise investment of these funds in public–academic and public–private partnerships can build wastewater analytic capacity and sustain implementation activities.

Although measuring levels of SARS-CoV-2 RNA in wastewater is relatively easy by some standards (in four hours we taught a wastewater treatment plant operator to do this with high fidelity), interpreting wastewater disease data is complex. The public health significance of a wastewater SARS-CoV-2 signal requires contextualization, an understanding of the limits of the approach, and further analysis of its correspondence with traditional disease surveillance metrics, such as hospitalization rates. Although Kotlarz et al. reported significant correlations between the wastewater and clinical signals during their study, there were also instances when these surveillance methods disagreed. As public health officials gain experience using wastewater data, it will be important to continue to evaluate wastewater's performance compared with traditional surveillance data sources, develop visualization and analytic tools to support its use, and provide opportunities for sharing best practices.

In summary, Kotlarz et al. and others have demonstrated the public health potential of wastewater testing, particularly in the context of the COVID-19 pandemic. The groundswell of enthusiasm in the research and public health sectors suggests that wastewater testing will continue to integrate with more established public health disease surveillance approaches. Although wastewater testing has challenges that inspire creative problem solving, we believe that its advantages make it a compelling tool for public health surveillance. AJPH

ACKNOWLEDGMENTS

The authors received support from the Office of the Director, National Institutes of Health (NIH; grant U01DA053903), the National Science Foundation (NSF; grant 2154934), and the Centers for Disease Control and Prevention (CDC; contract 75D30120C09531).

Note. The content of this editorial is solely the responsibility of the authors and does not necessarily represent the official views of the NIH, NSF, or the CDC.

CORRESPONDENCE

Correspondence should be sent to James Keck, 2195 Harrodsburg Rd, Ste 125, Lexington, KY 40504 (e-mail: James.Keck@uky.edu). Reprints can be ordered at http://www.ajph.org by clicking the "Reprints" link.

PUBLICATION INFORMATION

Full Citation: Keck JW, Berry SM. Wastewater surveillance—"messy" science with public health potential. *Am J Public Health.* 2023;113(1):6–8.

Acceptance Date: September 28, 2022.

DOI: https://doi.org/10.2105/AJPH.2022.307141

CONTRIBUTORS

The authors contributed equally to the conceptualization and writing of this editorial.

CONFLICTS OF INTEREST

S. M. Berry reports ownership interest in Salus Discovery LLC. J. W. Keck has no conflicts of interest to declare.

REFERENCES

1. COVID-19 WBE Collaborative. COVIDPoops19 dashboard. 2022. Available at: https://www.covid19wbec.org/covidpoops19. Accessed September 19, 2022.
2. Centers for Disease Control and Prevention. Using wastewater surveillance data to support the COVID-19 response—United States, 2020–2021. *MMWR Morb Mortal Wkly Rep.* 2021;70(36):1242–1244. https://doi.org/10.15585/mmwr.mm7036a2
3. Wright J, Driver EM, Bowes DA, Johnston B, Halden RU. Comparison of high-frequency in-pipe SARS-CoV-2 wastewater-based surveillance to concurrent COVID-19 random clinical testing on a public U.S. university campus. *Sci Total Environ.* 2022;820:152877. https://doi.org/10.1016/j.scitotenv.2021.152877
4. Cutrupi F, Cadonna M, Manara S, et al. The wave of the SARS-CoV-2 omicron variant resulted in a rapid spike and decline as highlighted by municipal wastewater surveillance. *Environ Technol Innov.* 2022;28:102667. https://doi.org/10.1016/j.eti.2022.102667
5. Daigle J, Racher K, Hazenberg J, et al. A sensitive and rapid wastewater test for SARS-COV-2 and its use for the early detection of a cluster of cases in a remote community. *Appl Environ Microbiol.* 2022;88(5):e01740-21. https://doi.org/10.1128/AEM.01740-21
6. Foladori P, Cutrupi F, Segata N, et al. SARS-CoV-2 from faeces to wastewater treatment: what do we know? A review. *Sci Total Environ.* 2020;743:140444. https://doi.org/10.1016/j.scitotenv.2020.140444
7. Brouwer AF, Eisenberg JNS, Pomeroy CD, et al. Epidemiology of the silent polio outbreak in Rahat, Israel, based on modeling of environmental surveillance data. *Proc Natl Acad Sci U S A.* 2018;115(45):E10625–E10633. https://doi.org/10.1073/pnas.1808798115
8. Centers for Disease Control and Prevention. Public health response to a case of paralytic poliomyelitis in an unvaccinated person and detection of poliovirus in wastewater—New York, June–August 2022. *MMWR Morb Mortal Wkly Rep.* 2022;71(33):1065–1068. https://doi.org/10.15585/mmwr.mm7133e2
9. Karthikeyan S, Levy JI, De Hoff P, et al. Wastewater sequencing reveals early cryptic SARS-CoV-2 variant transmission. *Nature.* 2022;609(7925):101–108. https://doi.org/10.1038/s41586-022-05049-6
10. Harrington A, Vo V, Papp K, et al. Urban monitoring of antimicrobial resistance during a COVID-19 surge through wastewater surveillance. *Sci Total Environ.* 2022;853:158577. https://doi.org/10.1016/j.scitotenv.2022.158577
11. Lemas DJ, Loop MS, Duong M, et al. Estimating drug consumption during a college sporting event from wastewater using liquid chromatography mass spectrometry. *Sci Total Environ.* 2021;764:143963. https://doi.org/10.1016/j.scitotenv.2020.143963
12. Kumar R, Adhikari S, Driver EM, et al. Towards a novel application of wastewater-based epidemiology in population-wide assessment of exposure to volatile organic compounds. *Sci Total Environ.* 2022;845:157008. https://doi.org/10.1016/j.scitotenv.2022.157008

Two Decades of Progress in Undergraduate Public Health: Where Do We Go From Here?

Richard K. Riegelman, MD, PhD, MPH

ABOUT THE AUTHOR

The author is with the Milken Institute School of Public Health, George Washington University, Washington, DC.

See also Leider et al., p. 115.

It has been two decades since the Institute of Medicine wrote that "all undergraduates should have access to education in public health."[1(p144)] This recommendation was aspirational. Nevertheless, it catalyzed a movement to develop undergraduate majors and minors in public health as well as extend public health education to community colleges, clinical health professionals, and an expanding audience of students domestically and globally.[2]

In their article in this issue of *AJPH*, Leider et al. (p. 115) report on the status of public health bachelor's degree education in the United States and provide useful data on the number of graduates, debt, and employment. As indicated in the article, undergraduate public health education has grown rapidly over the past two decades, with more than 18 000 bachelor's degrees conferred in 2020. There are now more bachelor's degrees granted each year than MPH degrees. As demonstrated in the article, the graduates reflect the racial and ethnic diversity that is needed in the future public health workforce.

The work of the past two decades has laid the groundwork for the future. Undergraduate public health education is now integrated into the fabric of bachelor's degree education not only in institutions with graduate public health education but also in what have been called "stand-alone" institutions that offer undergraduate public health majors but not graduate work.

The Council on Education for Public Health now accredits stand-alone programs as well as undergraduate programs as part of graduate programs and schools of public health.[3] The Association of Schools and Programs of Public Health has established the Undergraduate Network for Education in Public Health, which now includes more than 200 member institutions. The association sponsors an annual undergraduate public health conference that is open to network members as well as nonmembers.[4]

WHERE DO WE GO FROM HERE?

Now that undergraduate public health education is fully established in the mainstream of public health and undergraduate education, it is important to ask where undergraduate public health education goes from here. In particular, how can bachelor's degree graduates help fulfill the current and future needs of public health practice?

The data presented by Leider et al. indicate that bachelor's degree graduates are obtaining their first employment primarily in not-for-profit and for-profit institutions as opposed to governmental public health agencies. The COVID-19 pandemic provides an opportunity to increase the interest of undergraduates in the field of governmental public health because it has brought to national attention the enormous needs for governmental public health and provided strong justification for sustained investments.

The growth of undergraduate public health education provides an opening to integrate public health education into the development of a national public health system. For this to occur, it is important to ask the following question: What are the barriers and what are the opportunities?

The MPH has been the dominant public health degree for more than a century, and understandably many governmental public health positions require an MPH degree. This has been a barrier to bachelor's degree employment. A high priority in the near future is to better delineate the roles of bachelor's degree graduates and MPH graduates in governmental public health and reflect these differences, especially in entry-level job descriptions.

Key to the entry of undergraduate public health majors into the governmental public health workforce is the opportunity to gain experience in public health departments. In the past, these opportunities have been limited and often reserved for MPH students. In addition, new curricula aimed at the needs of public health practice can better connect academia and practice.

POTENTIAL FUTURE INITIATIVES

There are a number of collaborative initiatives in the next few years that could help move undergraduate public health education into a new phase that emphasizes the growth and development of the governmental public health workforce and continues to expand the reach of undergraduate public health education. Examples are as follows:

- Expansion and development of academic public health departments: academic health departments have great potential to serve the needs of public health practice as well as academia. A growing number have been developed and nurtured over the past two decades with the encouragement of the Council on Linkages Between Academia and Public Health Practice.[5] A broad initiative to increase participation by health departments and by a wide range of undergraduate and graduate students, along with a stable and increasing level of federal and local financial support, could be pivotal to the future development of a national public health system.
- Expansion of Centers for Disease Control and Prevention (CDC) fellowships to include undergraduates: expansion of CDC fellowships to fully include undergraduates would provide important opportunities for career development in governmental public health. It would also send an important message that undergraduate public health education is now a full-fledged partner in the future public health system.
- Development of certificate programs in areas of need: the needs of the public health workforce require new curricula in the form of free-standing certificates often linked to certification examinations. For instance, the CDC is developing the disease intervention specialist certification. Preparation for this certification can be facilitated by offering free-standing certificate curricula at community colleges and four-year institutions. Other areas of need such as public health information systems might also benefit from certificate programs.

THE FUTURE OF UNDERGRADUATE PUBLIC HEALTH EDUCATION

Accomplishing these goals will require collaboration from the full range of public health organizations, including the Association of Schools and Programs of Public Health, the American Public Health Association, the Association of State and Territorial Health Officials, the National Association of County and City Health Officials, and the Council on Linkages. It will be important to focus on the future of undergraduate public health education as these organizations take on the bigger issue of developing a national public health system. Distinguishing between bachelor's- and master's-degree requirements in entry-level job descriptions would be a good starting point because it would focus the attention of public health practice as well as academia on the need to connect bachelor's degree public health education with the needs of the public health workforce.

Leider et al. do an excellent job of bringing together degree conferral and employment data on bachelor's degrees. Unfortunately, parallel data on the broader educational impact of the undergraduate public health movement are not available.

Public health is increasingly becoming a core undergraduate discipline. The goal for all undergraduates to have access to education in public health has not been fully accomplished, but it is no longer aspirational. Extensive anecdotal experience strongly suggests that students from a wide range of majors are increasingly engaging in introductory public health coursework or pursuing a minor in public health. The interest in public health among nursing, medicine, pharmacy, and other clinical disciplines is growing rapidly. An additional reservoir of interest in public health education exists at the community college level, where the majority of students now come from minority populations, and coursework in public health is still very limited. The population health management movement is increasingly integrating public health principles into the delivery of health care to populations.[6]

The past two decades have demonstrated that fundamental educational change is possible as public health has increasingly been integrated throughout undergraduate education. The next two decades provide an opportunity to develop a national public health system with public health bachelor's degree and certificate graduates fully integrated into the emerging system. AJPH

CORRESPONDENCE

Correspondence should be sent to Richard K. Riegelman, MD, PhD, MPH, 950 New Hampshire Ave NW, Washington, DC 20052 (e-mail: rriegelman@gmail.com). Reprints can be ordered at http://www.ajph.org by clicking the "Reprints" link.

PUBLICATION INFORMATION

Full Citation: Riegelman RK. Two decades of progress in undergraduate public health: where do we go from here? *Am J Public Health*. 2023;113(1): 9–11.

Acceptance Date: October 2, 2022.

DOI: https://doi.org/10.2105/AJPH.2022.307145

CONFLICTS OF INTEREST

The author is a series editor and author in Jones and Bartlett Learning's Essential Public Health series.

REFERENCES

1. Institute of Medicine. *The Future of the Public's Health in the 21st Century*. Washington, DC: National Academy Press; 2003.
2. Riegelman RK, Albertine S, Wykoff R. A history of undergraduate education for public health: from behind the scenes to center stage. *Front Public Health*. 2015;3:70. https://doi.org/10.3389/fpubh.2015.00070
3. Council on Education for Public Health. Stand-alone baccalaureate programs. Available at: https://media.ceph.org/documents/2018.SBP criteria.pdf. Accessed September 9, 2022.
4. Association of Schools and Programs of Public Health. Undergraduate network for education in public health. Available at: https://aspph.org/membership/undergraduate-network. Accessed September 9, 2022.
5. Council on Linkages Between Academia and Public Health Practice. Academic health department learning community. Available at: http://www.phf.org/programs/AHDLC/Pages/Academic_Health_Department_Learning_Community.aspx. Accessed September 9, 2022.
6. American Hospital Association. Population health management. Available at: https://www.aha.org/center/population-health-management. Accessed September 9, 2022.

Environmental Justice From Pennsylvania to Paris: A Public Health of Consequence, January 2023

Farzana Kapadia, PhD, MPH

ABOUT THE AUTHOR

Farzana Kapadia is deputy editor of AJPH *and is with the School of Global Public Health, New York University, New York, NY.*

See also Schmeltz et al., p. 15.

Mitigating the impact of environmental disasters and climate change on vulnerable groups of people calls for an environmental justice–based approach that makes "the fair treatment and meaningful involvement of all people regardless of race, color, national origin, or income" a top priority.[1] In 2011, Gracia and Koh presciently wrote that promoting environmental justice "requires reaffirming, revitalizing, and reinvigorating past national commitments" to how we plan and sustain laws, policies, and practices.[2(pS14)] An environmental justice–based approach to ensuring "greater access to health care, clean air and water, healthy and affordable food, community capacity building through grants and technical assistance, and training to educate the health workforce about environmentally associated health conditions"[2(pS15)] for all is the path to bridging environmental justice and health equity.[3] In this editorial, I highlight the historical and current calls for an environmental justice approach to preparing for and responding to man-made as well as natural environmental disasters.

DONORA, PENNSYLVANIA

Ask now, and it is unlikely that many people know where Donora, Pennsylvania, is or what it signifies. In late October 1948, a heavy smog rising from steel and zinc factories enveloped Donora and caused at least 20 deaths and close to 6000 mild and moderate cases of respiratory distress immediately after the smog settled.[4] The preliminary US Public Health Service (USPHS) report on the immediate impacts of the Donora smog pointed to increased mortality and morbidity among the elderly and those with preexisting cardiopulmonary conditions.[5] Adding to these findings, a follow-up study provided evidence of the unequal distribution of mortality and morbidity—those who were poor, not White, of limited English proficiency, and living in substandard housing were overrepresented among the dead and the ill immediately after the smog and during follow-up investigations.[6]

Today we recognize what happened in Donora as an example of environmental injustice in which the commercial concerns of the steel and zinc industries superseded concerns about the health and well-being of factory workers. Moreover, without any federal oversight, these industries were able to operate factories with little to no regulatory oversight.

While Donora was most certainly not the only man-made environmental disaster in the United States during this time, it stands out for being a driving force behind the enactment of the federal Clean Air Act in 1963. The Clean Air Act was the first federal legislation concerned with "controlling" air pollution and authorized the USPHS to support research into techniques for monitoring and controlling air pollution. As Vernon MacKenzie,[7] chief of the Division of Air Pollution in the USPHS, wrote,

> Air pollution can no longer be dismissed with excuses and half-way measures. Through the congressional action in enacting the Clean Air Act, we have made a commitment to bring an end to the steady increase in the national air pollution problem. We must keep that commitment.[7(p904)]

PLANNING, PREVENTING, AND RESPONDING

Fast forward and, according to the National Oceanic and Atmospheric Administration, Hurricane Ian was the 15th environmental disaster to cause at least $1 billion in damage as of October 11, 2022 (https://bit.ly/3yKUAzY). To date, more than 100 people have died in Florida as a result of the hurricane, making it the deadliest hurricane to hit

AJPH January 2023, Vol 113, No. 1

Florida in more than 85 years (https://bit.ly/3eCRAiw). One of the questions that will likely be raised in the months to come is whether local preparedness as well as response were appropriate and implemented in a timely manner.

Such questions are of greater relevance now, and as Schmeltz et al. (p. 15) write about in this issue of *AJPH*, there are indeed gaps in preparing for and responding to climate change hazards. While their article focuses on extreme heat events, the findings are applicable to a range of extreme weather events and environmental disasters. Their review of Heat Action Plans in California suggests that the current planning focuses on emergency response and warrants redirection to focus on preventing negative health outcomes. A review of the organization and governance of extant Heat Action Plans in California also indicates a greater need to focus on preparedness for extreme heat events as well as coordinating with local and state departments of health to devise a public health preparedness plan and response.

Health departments and local stakeholders are needed to foster environmental justice and protect vulnerable people.[8] The need for such coordination is supported by Schwarz et al., who found that people experiencing homelessness and were either younger or elderly or had an underlying mental health burden were especially vulnerable to heat waves and more likely to seek care in an emergency department for health care during extreme heat events.[9] Planning and practice that seeks to ensure resources are equitably allocated to those most likely to experience greatest exposure to environmental harms is necessary to ensure health equity and environmental justice.[10]

HOW MUCH DOES 1.5°C REALLY MATTER?

As confirmed by the International Panel on Climate Change's Special Report on Global Warming, a 1.5°C (2.7°F for those in the United States) increase in the average global temperature will cause an escalation of natural environmental disasters across the world.[11] This increase will yield more extreme weather in the forms of heat waves and polar vortexes, more and longer periods of droughts, worsening floods and heavy rains, decreased availability of fresh water, rising sea levels, and shrinking polar ice caps. The list is long, and the consequence of each one of these environmental disasters threatens the security of our global community, particularly for those with the fewest resources and in the most vulnerable situations. This past year alone, we witnessed large wildfires and severe heat waves across the United States and Europe; flooding in Bangladesh, India, Pakistan, Brazil, and in the Appalachian (Kentucky) region in the United States; and another above-average hurricane and tropical storm season in the Atlantic region.

UPHOLDING OUR OBLIGATION TO THE PARIS ACCORDS

With the Clean Air Act of 1963, the creation of the Environmental Protection Agency (EPA) in 1970, and the Paris Accords of 2015, there were slow but steady efforts to motivate state, federal, and global actions to reduce greenhouse gas emissions and slow increases in global temperatures to achieve a climate-neutral world by 2050. In affirming the 1963 commitment to bringing an end to the "national air pollution problem," in 2015, the Obama administration issued a broad and comprehensive Clean Power Plan under the Clean Air Act to rein in power plant emissions and provide states opportunities to identify and implement plans to switch to cleaner energy options. Under the Trump administration, the vast majority of rules enumerated in the Clean Power Plan were rolled back (https://nyti.ms/3galYA0). And while the Biden administration has sought to undo these reversals, in some instances, it may take years to fully undo these rollbacks.

Most recently, the US Supreme Court ruled in *West Virginia v. Environmental Protection Agency* (EPA) that the EPA could not put state-level caps on carbon emissions as clearly laid out in the 1970 Clean Air Act, but that this authority rested with the US Congress. In so ruling, the Court opined that the EPA lacked the authority to pursue its primary mission of limiting pollution attributable to toxic and harmful substances and lacked authority to pursue goals set under the Clean Power Plan.

POLICIES, NOT POLITICS

The *West Virginia v. EPA* ruling poses significant threats to our ability to meet our obligations to the Paris Accords and the global community to reduce our greenhouse gas emissions and slow the climate crisis. For the public health community, this ruling threatens progress in achieving health equity as well as in promoting environmental justice and ignores the substantial evidence base on the physical and mental health harms associated with environmental disasters. So, this editorial serves as a call to all in the public health community to advocate and agitate for climate justice, for environmental justice and health equality for all of humanity.

In the words of Jake Edwards of the Onondaga Nation Council of Chiefs: "We all need the same things: clean air and clean water. We have a lot of work to do, but if we can combine our strengths, we can fight for what's right" (https://bit.ly/3VLwejM). AJPH

CORRESPONDENCE

Correspondence should be sent to Farzana Kapadia, PhD, MPH, New York University, School of Global Public Health, 708 Broadway, Room 729, New York, NY 10003 (e-mail: farzana.kapadia@nyu.edu). Reprints can be ordered at https://ajph.org by clicking the "Reprints" link.

PUBLICATION INFORMATION

Full Citation: Kapadia F. Environmental justice from Pennsylvania to Paris: a public health of consequence, January 2023. *Am J Public Health*. 2023;113(1):12–14.

Acceptance Date: October 18, 2022.

DOI: https://doi.org/10.2105/AJPH.2022.307156

CONFLICTS OF INTEREST

The author has no conflicts of interest to disclose.

REFERENCES

1. US Environmental Protection Agency. Environmental justice. Available at: https://www.epa.gov/environmentaljustice. Accessed October 15, 2022.
2. Gracia JN, Koh HK. Promoting environmental justice. *Am J Public Health*. 2011;101(suppl 1):S14–S16. https://doi.org/10.2105/AJPH.2011.300406
3. Ruffin J. A renewed commitment to environmental justice in health disparities research. *Am J Public Health*. 2011;101(suppl 1):S12–S14. https://doi.org/10.2105/AJPH.2011.300480
4. Jacobs ET, Burgess JL, Abbott MB. The Donora smog revisited: 70 years after the event that inspired the Clean Air Act. *Am J Public Health*. 2018;108(suppl 2):S85–S88. https://doi.org/10.2105/AJPH.2017.304219
5. Townsend JG. Investigation of the smog incident in Donora, Pa., and vicinity. *Am J Public Health Nations Health*. 1950;40(2):183–189. https://doi.org/10.2105/AJPH.40.2.183
6. Ciocco A, Thompson DJ. A follow-up of Donora ten years after: methodology and findings. *Am J Public Health Nations Health*. 1961;51(2):155–164. https://doi.org/10.2105/AJPH.51.2.155
7. MacKenzie VG. The Clean Air Act and its implications. *Am J Public Health Nations Health*. 1965;55(6):901–904. https://doi.org/10.2105/AJPH.55.6.901
8. Schmeltz MT. Climate change is already exacerbating current social inequities. *Am J Public Health*. 2021;111(1):10–11. https://doi.org/10.2105/AJPH.2020.306010
9. Schwarz L, Castillo EM, Chan TC, et al. Heat waves and emergency department visits among the homeless, San Diego, 2012–2019. *Am J Public Health*. 2022;112(1):98–106. https://doi.org/10.2105/AJPH.2021.306557
10. Carrión D, Belcourt A, Fuller CH. Heading upstream: strategies to shift environmental justice research from disparities to equity. *Am J Public Health*. 2022;112(1):59–62. https://doi.org/10.2105/AJPH.2021.306605
11. International Panel on Climate Change. Summary for policymakers. In: Masson-Delmotte V, Zhai P, Pörtner HO, et al., eds. *Global Warming of 1.5°C. An IPCC Special Report on the Impacts of Global Warming of 1.5°C Above Pre-industrial Levels and Related Global Greenhouse Gas Emission Pathways, in the Context of Strengthening the Global Response to the Threat of Climate Change, Sustainable Development, and Efforts to Eradicate Poverty.* Cambridge, UK, and New York, NY: Cambridge University Press; 2018:3–24.

Extreme Heat Governance: A Critical Analysis of Heat Action Plans in California

Michael T. Schmeltz, DrPH, MS, Jason A. Smith, JD, MTS, Isabella Olmos, BS, and Erin Quintero, BS

ABOUT THE AUTHORS

Michael T. Schmeltz is with the Department of Public Health, California State University, East Bay, Hayward. Jason A. Smith is with the College of Health and Human Development, California State University, Fullerton. Isabella Olmos and Erin Quintero are recent graduates from the Department of Public Health, California State University, East Bay.

See also Kapadia, p. 12.

Extreme heat events have adverse effects on population health, causing heat-related illnesses, such as heat exhaustion and heat stroke, but also exacerbating underlying medical conditions, such as cardiac and respiratory diseases, through various mechanisms.[1] In the United States, from 2000 to 2010 there were approximately 28 000 recorded heat-related hospitalizations, and between 2004 and 2018, an average of about 700 people died because of heat-related illnesses, making heat the deadliest weather-related hazard in the United States.[2,3] These figures do not represent heat morbidity and mortality that were not attributable by *International Classification of Diseases* (Geneva, Switzerland: World Health Organization) *Ninth Revision* (1980) or *10th Revision* (1992) code to a confirmed diagnosis of heat-related illnesses, which likely results in underreporting.[4] Additionally, the health consequences of extreme heat are amplified by sociodemographic vulnerabilities and our built environment. As extreme heat events continue to increase in frequency and intensity, individuals, communities, and the municipalities in which they live will need to prepare and adapt.

Health impacts from high ambient temperatures have led many municipalities to develop plans to respond to extreme heat events. These plans are sometimes referred to as excessive heat emergency plans, heat-health response plans, or heat action plans (HAPs). Many European countries implemented HAPs following the 2003 European heat wave.[5] In the United States, a number of cities have developed HAPs,[6,7] although the vast majority of US cities and regions rely only on local National Weather Service offices to issue heat advisories based on heat index forecasts that may not be linked to local HAPs.[8]

In 2020, the US Centers for Disease Control and Prevention (CDC) released a technical report on the summary and strategies for HAPs and ascribed their focus to emergency response planning or long-term planning for extreme heat. The report identifies that plans can stand alone or be an annex to an all-hazards plan and specifically identifies emergency preparedness and management activities when coordinating plans.[9] Although the CDC report is not a step-by-step guide or an all-inclusive approach to how to specifically prepare or coordinate a HAP, the reference to emergency operations plans and the location of HAPs in all-hazards mitigation plans suggest that extreme heat is an event that consistently requires an emergency response and is best understood in that context. However, climate change will increase the likelihood and frequency of extreme weather events, such as extreme heat, and these events have increased substantially over the past decades and will continue to affect regions of the globe regularly.[10] We argue that the increasing frequency and regularity of these events move them from emergencies to an issue to be planned for with preventive health plans.

Since the terrorist attacks of September 11, 2001, the public health legal frameworks that emphasized preparedness have shifted to a concept that emphasized emergencies. This framing emphasizes an emergency as an event that overwhelms the capacity of the health care system.[11] One of the defining characteristics of an emergency is its unpredictability or its unforeseeability. Given that these events will be more frequent, the health and public health systems must move the approach to extreme heat events from emergency to more traditional public health governance structures, usually located in departments of public health or in close coordination. This move supports two very important conceptual shifts. First, it situates the effects of the climate crisis more clearly in the regular governance structures of the state as a long-term policy consideration. Second, it supports the transition of our public health care systems to a climate-resilient model. Keeping the frameworks entirely in offices of emergency services

AJPH January 2023, Vol 113, No. 1

abrogates the duty of the state to grapple with the climate crisis as a long-term reality.

Public health departments can be ideal partners and leaders in addressing climate and health issues, particularly those at the local jurisdiction. They are usually the designated government agency that is tasked with protecting the health of communities, are a trusted voice with close ties to the communities they serve, and have a proven ability to confront and overcome complex health issues, such as climate change.[12] Guidance on HAPs is not new but has not been implemented equally across regions. Additionally, even information about extreme heat on local and regional government Web sites can be sparse, and coverage is not always the same.[13]

We used local public health jurisdictions in California to examine how HAPs are organized and implemented to protect populations from the health impacts of extreme heat. We argue that extreme heat events should be in the jurisdiction of public health response and that these organizations are key to leading or closely supporting efforts to reduce the health impacts associated with extreme heat.

EXAMINATION OF HEAT ACTION PLANS

To examine the current governance structure of HAPs, we conducted a desk review between August and December 2021 that focused on collecting publicly available written HAPs in California. We defined a "public health jurisdiction" as the lowest level of jurisdiction with public health authority in the state. California has 61 public health jurisdictions; 58 of these are run by a county and three are run by a city.

We conducted online searches using the same keywords for each public health jurisdiction (county/city name + heat plan and/or extreme heat; county/city name + excessive heat emergency; county/city name + extreme weather). We performed searches in Google and on county Web sites with search functions. We gathered and stored Web site links and copies of plans. When the online search did not yield any results, we contacted departments of public health and emergency services to request written plans. We included a plan when (1) a government agency issued it at the public health jurisdiction level, and (2) it was a standalone HAP, or the response to extreme heat was a main topic in a multihazard plan (e.g., California's Local Hazard Mitigation Plan). We did not include public health jurisdictions that did not have an available plan online or that did not respond to our request, under the assumption that a written plan was not publicly available.

We developed a checklist of core elements for HAPs based on previously developed guidelines. The checklist was influenced mainly by the World Health Organization's "Heat-Health Action Plans: Guidance" but also included criteria to reflect recent reviews of HAPs; improvements in climate surveillance, monitoring, and forecasting; specific needs for vulnerable populations; and effective communication of heat-health information.[7,9,14–18] The checklist consisted of nine core elements that we identified as important for a successful HAP:

1. An identified lead body to coordinate HAP with clear guidance on heat-risk governance;
2. An accurate (to locality) heat-health warning system, including threshold for action based on local health data;
3. Identification and outreach plans (communication and intervention) specifically targeted to vulnerable populations;
4. A communication guide for heat-related health information, including general public education and awareness campaigns with an emphasis on health behavior and health promotion;
5. Preparedness for social and health systems, including staffing capacity, infrastructure, and health care, including specific procedures for emergency medical services, hospitals, nursing homes, and caretakers of vulnerable populations;
6. Strategies for short- and medium-term reduction in indoor heat exposure, including passive and active cooling;
7. Long-term planning addressing urban design and building, energy, and transportation policies that reduce heat exposure and projections of future changes in heat morbidity and mortality from shifting demographics and societal conditions;
8. Real-term (syndromic) surveillance of heat-health outcomes for emergency and rapid response, including coordination between responding agencies; and
9. An evaluation of the HAP, including a comprehensive set of metrics for evaluation and evidence of effectiveness.

Our review of HAPs in California identified 37 (60%) public health jurisdictions with at least one core element identified in the plans. Of these, 24 (65%) jurisdictions had one to three core elements identified, and only seven (19%) jurisdictions had four or more core elements identified. We were unable to identify or access a HAP for 24 public health jurisdictions (Figure A, available as a supplement to the online version of this article at http://www.ajph.org). Of all the plans we identified, no plans were located in departments of public health. We gathered all plans from either county government Web sites or the county agency dedicated to emergency management.

Even with plans partially completed, many of the core elements provided limited information. For example, all plans that contained core element 2—comprehensive heat-health warning systems—only included information from National Weather Services' advisories or used the National Weather Services' HeatRisk tool. There was no evidence that plans reviewed local epidemiological data in the development of location-specific heat-health warning systems for their communities. Similarly, plans that were partially completed were addenda or annexes to local hazard mitigation plans, which included information on populations that were generally vulnerable to severe weather hazards, including extreme heat.

Approximately 12 (32%) plans included a description of a "lead body" and some form of "communication plan" to get messages to the public concerning extreme heat events—either before or during the event. Few plans identified ways they specifically "prepared key stakeholders" or identified "short- and medium-term strategies" or "long-term strategies" for reducing exposure to extreme heat in their jurisdiction. There was no evidence that any HAPs contained information regarding "real-time surveillance."

CONCLUSIONS

Anthropogenic climate change and its consequences are often described as an emergency or crisis, particularly when it comes to the impacts on public health and the exacerbation of social and health inequities.[19] We are not discounting the use of the word "emergency" when describing the threat of global climate change. It implies correctly that urgent action is needed to address the human health impacts of climate change.[20] The action, however, is not to avoid the disruptions of anthropogenic climate change but to prepare for them and to manage them as an ongoing characteristic of life in the Anthropocene. The emergency is a collective failure to act, not the extreme heat. Our overall objective is to start to better determine and clarify the policies and governance structures that we can use to accomplish an effective adaptation and to identify gaps that require fundamental changes to governance structures and laws to reduce the magnitude of and prepare for climate hazards, such as extreme heat.

Previous studies examining HAPs have done so at the municipal level,[7,21,22] with mixed results, and others have been assessed at the national, state, or regional level.[15,16,23] These studies emphasize the large variability in how HAPs are implemented and assessed at various levels of governance and the ad hoc approach to the issue. High ambient temperatures and extreme heat events are explicitly linked to negative public health outcomes. Although the effects of extreme heat can affect multiple sectors of society, it is the effect on human health and the infrastructure that supports human health that is of primary concern. Public health departments are key to assessing population health, creating policies and plans, and improving health outcomes. Heat-related illnesses associated with extreme heat are preventable, and human health is a unifying organizing principle for considering the impacts of extreme heat and organizing planning for it. We recommend that the governance structure of HAPs focus on the health implications of extreme heat events, as health outcomes are strongly tied to local health department activities and missions and are equipped to coordinate responses over the long term and coordinate closely with emergency management to address immediate responses to extreme heat events.

We acknowledge that the ongoing COVID-19 pandemic has highlighted significant gaps in our public health infrastructure. Climate change is a current and long-term crisis that will further exacerbate structural weaknesses in our public health system and will need significant investment and resources to overcome. To achieve this, programs such as the CDC's Building Resilience Against Climate Effects and the workforce capacity–building Climate Corps can better fund and staff public health agencies to address climate and health issues. This transition from an emergency framing to a public health framing cannot be an abrupt one, as the Intergovernmental Panel on Climate Change has identified in its most recent report on mitigation that the transitions involved in climate adaptation and mitigation will produce tensions and raise justice and equity concerns that must be managed.[24] This requires planning, consensus building, and a clear understanding of context. Emergency operations and management will still need to coordinate and respond to the immediate needs of the community, but preparation and preventive measures through departments of public health will be key to building resilience in communities to future extreme heat events.

In addition, although we identify vulnerability assessment and outreach plans in the core elements of a HAP, we should note that developing plans is one part of the process; community engagement and implementation are other important factors in HAP effectiveness. Health departments have experience in including communities in planning; public health frameworks' reliance on the social determinants of health and health equity makes public health a natural location for this coordination activity.

To achieve results in governance related to extreme heat in California, coordination among various stakeholders will be needed—no individual or single agency can achieve this alone. In a recent report highlighting adaptation to extreme heat in California, one of the first priority policies the authors identified was a lack of central authority providing coordination, technical assistance, and strategic funding to address extreme heat. Los Angeles, California, recently appointed a chief heat officer, and there is current (as of this writing) legislation in California, AB-2076, that will establish the statewide Extreme Heat and Community Resilience Program.

Departments of public health should be prioritized and provided with strategic funding for technical assistance in addressing the health concerns of extreme heat. Another priority policy identified that local hazard planning, such as local hazard mitigation plans, are likely not preparing municipalities to address extreme heat in their communities.[25] Although local hazard mitigation plans are not emergency preparedness plans, many of the elements of HAPs can be found there. There should be a clear distinction between emergency disaster preparedness and public health preparedness, with the latter emphasizing prevention and preparedness in public health agencies to support or lead efforts in developing successful HAPs.

Some limitations of our review stem from information bias on the availability of HAPs and the use of local hazard mitigation plans and other emergency preparedness plans as proxies for HAPs. We acknowledge that health departments are not currently resourced to play this role and that there are significant legal, political, and governance issues that need to be explored and resolved. We urge public health law and policy scholars and practitioners to begin this urgent work. Public health departments can be a natural home for this work. Public health has a strong commitment to health equity, employs population perspectives and systems thinking in its work, and has experience working in communities. Our analysis of HAPs in California makes clear that the ad hoc approach to this issue is not working and that leadership at the state and regional levels is required. AJPH

CORRESPONDENCE

Correspondence should be sent to Michael T. Schmeltz, Assistant Professor, California State University, East Bay, SF502, 25800 Carlos Bee Blvd, Hayward, CA 94542 (e-mail: michael.schmeltz@csueastbay.edu). Reprints can be ordered at http://www.ajph.org by clicking the "Reprints" link.

PUBLICATION INFORMATION

Full Citation: Schmeltz MT, Smith JA, Olmos I, Quintero E. Extreme heat governance: a critical analysis of heat action plans in California. *Am J Public Health*. 2023;113(1):15–19.

Acceptance Date: August 30, 2022.

DOI: https://doi.org/10.2105/AJPH.2022.307117

CONTRIBUTORS

M. T. Schmeltz and J. A. Smith developed the study concept and design and drafted the article. M. T. Schmeltz, I. Olmos, and E. Quintero collected and analyzed the data. All authors interpreted the data and contributed to the final draft of the article.

CONFLICTS OF INTEREST

The authors have no conflicts of interest to declare.

REFERENCES

1. Li M, Gu S, Bi P, Yang J, Liu Q. Heat waves and morbidity: current knowledge and further direction—a comprehensive literature review. *Int J Environ Res Public Health*. 2015;12(5):5256–5283. https://doi.org/10.3390/ijerph120505256
2. Centers for Disease Control and Prevention. Heat stress illness hospitalizations—environmental public health tracking program, 20 states, 2001–2010. *MMWR Surveill Summ*. 2014;63(13):1–10.
3. Centers for Disease Control and Prevention. Heat-related deaths—United States, 2004–2018. *MMWR Morb Mortal Wkly Rep*. 2020;69(24):729–734. https://doi.org/10.15585/mmwr.mm6924a1
4. Schmeltz MT, Sembajwe G, Marcotullio PJ, Grassman JA, Himmelstein DU, Woolhandler S. Identifying individual risk factors and documenting the pattern of heat-related illness through analyses of hospitalization and patterns of household cooling. *PLoS One*. 2015;10(3):e0118958. https://doi.org/10.1371/journal.pone.0118958.
5. Robine JM, Cheung SL, Le Roy S, et al. Death toll exceeded 70,000 in Europe during the summer of 2003. *C R Biol*. 2008;331(2):171–178. https://doi.org/10.1016/j.crvi.2007.12.001
6. Kalkstein AJ, Sheridan SC. The social impacts of the heat–health watch/warning system in Phoenix, Arizona: assessing the perceived risk and response of the public. *Int J Biometeorol*. 2007;52(1):43–55. https://doi.org/10.1007/s00484-006-0073-4
7. Benmarhnia T, Schwarz L, Nori-Sarma A, Bell ML. Quantifying the impact of changing the threshold of New York City heat emergency plan in reducing heat-related illnesses. *Environ Res Lett*. 2019;14(11):114006. https://doi.org/10.1088/1748-9326/ab402e
8. Weinberger KR, Zanobetti A, Schwartz J, Wellenius GA. Effectiveness of National Weather Service heat alerts in preventing mortality in 20 US cities. *Environ Int*. 2018;116:30–38. https://doi.org/10.1016/j.envint.2018.03.028
9. Centers for Disease Control and Prevention. Heat response plans: summary of evidence and strategies for collaboration and implementation. January 31, 2020. Available at: https://stacks.cdc.gov/view/cdc/93705. Accessed October 26, 2022.
10. US Environmental Protection Agency. Climate change indicators: heat waves. July 2022. Available at: https://www.epa.gov/climate-indicators/climate-change-indicators-heat-waves. Accessed January 21, 2022.
11. Smith JA. Public health, governance, and the Anthropocene. *Houst J Health Law Policy*. 2018;18:169–202.
12. Rudolph L, Harrison C, Buckley L, North S. Climate change, health, and equity: a guide for local health departments. 2018. Available at: https://www.apha.org/topics-and-issues/climate-change/guide. Accessed January 25, 2022.
13. Zottarelli LK, Blake SA, Garza MT. Communicating heat-health information to the public: assessing municipal government extreme heat event website

content. *Weather Clim Soc.* 2022;14(1):311–321. https://doi.org/10.1175/WCAS-D-21-0019.1
14. Matthies F, Bickler G, Cardeñosa Marín N, Hales S. Heat-health action plans: guidance. 2008. Available at: http://www.euro.who.int/__data/assets/pdf_file/0006/95919/E91347.pdf. Accessed February 25, 2022.
15. McGregor GR, Bessemoulin P, Ebi KL, Menne B. Heatwaves and health: guidance on warning-system development. 2015. Available at: https://public.wmo.int/en/resources/library/heatwaves-and-health-guidance-warning-system-development. Accessed February 25, 2022.
16. Casanueva A, Burgstall A, Kotlarski S, et al. Overview of existing heat-health warning systems in Europe. *Int J Environ Res Public Health.* 2019;16(15):2657. https://doi.org/10.3390/ijerph16152657
17. Martinez GS, Linares C, Ayuso A, et al. Heat-health action plans in Europe: challenges ahead and how to tackle them. *Environ Res.* 2019;176:108548. https://doi.org/10.1016/j.envres.2019.108548
18. Ebi KL. Effective heat action plans: research to interventions. *Environ Res Lett.* 2019;6;14(12):122001. https://doi.org/10.1088/1748-9326/ab5ab0
19. Schmeltz MT. Climate change is already exacerbating current social inequities. *Am J Public Health.* 2021;111(1):10–11. https://doi.org/10.2105/AJPH.2020.306010
20. Henson B. Emergency, crisis, existential threat: the evolving lingo of climate change. November 2, 2021. Available at: https://yaleclimateconnections.org/2021/11/emergency-crisis-existential-threat-the-evolving-lingo-of-climate-change. Accessed March 2, 2022.
21. Sheehan MC, Khudairi F, Swaich GS, Hines W, Mehta S, Fox MA. Urban climate-health governance: charting the role of public health in large global city adaptation plans. *PLoS Climate.* 2022;1(3):e0000012. https://doi.org/10.1371/journal.pclm.0000012
22. M. French E, Hondula D, Turner K. How are US cities planning for heat? *DesignSafe-CI.* 2021. Available at: https://www.designsafe-ci.org/data/browser/public/designsafe.storage.published/PRJ-3180. Accessed October 26, 2022. https://doi.org/10.17603/ds2-xc9j-3054
23. Kotharkar R, Ghosh A. Progress in extreme heat management and warning systems: a systematic review of heat-health action plans (1995–2020). *Sustain Cities Soc.* 2022;76:103487. https://doi.org/10.1016/j.scs.2021.103487
24. Dubash NK, Mitchell C, Boasson EL, et al. National and sub-national policies and institutions. In Shukla PR, Skea J, Slade R, et al., eds. *Climate Change 2022: Mitigation of Climate Change. Working Group III Contribution to the IPCC Sixth Assessment Report.* Cambridge, UK: Cambridge University Press; 2022. https://doi.org/10.1017/9781009157926.015
25. DeShazo JR, Lim L, Pierce G. Adapting to extreme heat in California: assessing gaps in state-level policies and funding opportunities. 2021. Available at: https://innovation.luskin.ucla.edu/wp-content/uploads/2021/10/Adapting-to-Extreme-Heat-in-California.pdf. Accessed March 5, 2022.

Rethinking "Herd" Mentalities and Rethinking the Value of the History of Public Health

Jacob Steere-Williams, PhD

ABOUT THE AUTHOR

Jacob Steere-Williams is an associate professor of history and director of medical humanities at the College of Charleston in Charleston, SC. He also is the president of the Waring Library Society at the Medical University of South Carolina and associate editor of The Journal of the History of Medicine and Allied Sciences.

AJPH January 2023, Vol 113, No. 1

The COVID-19 pandemic continues to reveal the uneasy ways in which the public co-opts epidemiological terms about the incidence and spread of disease—sometimes unknowingly and unwittingly, sometimes nefariously. The latest social variant of this infectious cultural trait is the term "endemic," which started to appear in popular discourse in late 2021 and gained steam in the first half of 2022. To politicians, the mainstream media, and many everyday people, reframing COVID-19 as endemic was a linguistic and rhetorical magic bullet that might bring some relief. The pandemic could be relabeled, they believed, as something less virulent, less deadly. Or at least as something that was not talked about as much.

THE "PUBLIC VIEW" OF PUBLIC HEALTH

In the past few months, the term endemic has come to equate to normalcy, but not without significant pushback. Professional epidemiologists, evolutionary biologists, and historians of epidemiology, myself included, have cautioned against the endemic framing of COVID-19 on two fronts. On one hand, the global epidemiological data on the disease do not indicate a shift to widely regarded definitions of endemicity. The term endemicity also has colonial roots of being a tool to assign moral blame to the Global South and absolve governmental responsibility of pandemic preparedness and response.[1] Endemicity, in other words, is a shifty and shifting term, one with a powerful history.

While public health practitioners have decried the misplaced popular use of terms such as endemicity, historians, philosophers, and sociologists of science have not been entirely surprised, though they, too, sought flat-footed ways of theorizing the pandemic in early 2020.[2] Endemicity is only the latest wedge in the cultural milieu of epidemic negotiations between science and society and suggests that now, more than ever, we collectively need a more nuanced understanding of the history of disease concepts in epidemiology and public health. Early in the COVID-19 pandemic, both the public and public health practitioners turned to the history of past pandemics, particularly the 1918–1919 influenza pandemic. Some hoped to find, in this shallow leveling of past and present, patterns and structures to use in real-time health policy, while others, I am convinced, turned to the past for pandemic therapy. Most quickly lost interest.

THE SOCIAL ORIGINS OF "HERD IMMUNITY"

Much more fruitful is the rich historical analysis provided by Warwick Anderson in a recently published essay for *AJPH's* "Then and Now" section, titled, "Immunities of the Herd in Peace, War, and COVID-19."[3] In this provocative piece, Anderson calls for a rethinking of a ubiquitous and contentious term used during the past two and a half years—"herd immunity." Wielded early in the COVID-19 pandemic by libertarian groups and some far-right politicians in the Global North, pursuing herd immunity meant minimal governmental containment strategies, which would elicit herd immunity in populations through natural infection. As Anderson shows, there was significant pushback to the notion of herd immunity in the first half of 2020, particularly from scientists and public health officials who called the strategy, as virologist William Haseltine implored, "another word for mass murder."[4]

Reading Anderson's essay reminds us that the collective trauma of the past two years means that most of us have forgotten the intensity of the debate around herd immunity in 2020. This alone makes the essay a significant contribution to *AJPH*. But Anderson's essay does much more, penetrating into the heart of the history of the modern discipline of epidemiology to show how the concept of herd immunity emerged in early 20th century Britain and was deeply imbued with ideas not just from ecology and veterinary medicine, the obvious link to the concept of "herd," but also from social psychology, particularly the notion of altruism.

The term herd immunity was coined in 1923 by British experimental epidemiologists W. W. C. Topley and G. S. Wilson and further developed by Sheldon F. Dudley's studies of communal immunity in schoolchildren, as Anderson traces in the essay. But the term did not just emerge out of changes in academic epidemiology in the 1920s and 1930s. Instead, it borrowed from the social sciences, particularly William Trotter's theories of altruism. Herd immunity, Anderson demonstrates, meant almost the opposite in the mid-20th century to how it was weaponized in early 2020.

WHAT CAN THE HISTORY OF EPIDEMIOLOGY OFFER?

Anderson's powerful essay is the kind of analysis and insight that will arm readers of *AJPH* with the tools for understanding and engaging with the history of epidemiology in public discourse. Devoid of incoherent neologism and denying a familiar approach to the history of epidemiology that ignores complexity and embraces heroic "founders" and "moments," Anderson's approach is a stark reminder that we need to dramatically rethink the value of the history of epidemiology in public discussion and in public health practice today. This is particularly true of the rich and complicated set of developments in professional Anglo-American epidemiology that occurred in the first half of the 20th century. The fairytale histories of epidemiology routinely taught in undergraduate textbooks and classrooms serve mostly to reify what Olga Amsterdamska called "demarcating" the professional boundaries of epidemiology."[5] As Anderson's essay suggests, we can, and we should, be doing a lot more than disciplinary policing.

The COVID-19 pandemic has thrown professional epidemiologists and the discipline of epidemiology into the public spotlight in ways few could have predicted before January 2020. In the process, it has also revealed the dangerous ways with which the public employs epidemiological terms and the uneasiness with which popular ideas persist in the history of the field. Anderson's foray into the past and present—the "Then and Now" at the heart of *AJPH*—of herd immunity will hopefully inspire further rethinking of the history of epidemiology and, in the process, help us to more effectively communicate the key concepts of epidemiology to broad public audiences and policymakers. AJPH

CORRESPONDENCE

Correspondence may be sent to Jacob Steere-Williams, Department of History, College of Charleston, 66 George St, Charleston, SC 29424 (e-mail: steerewilliamsj@cofc.edu). Reprints can be ordered at https://ajph.org by clicking the "Reprints" link.

PUBLICATION INFORMATION

Full Citation: Steere-Williams J. Rethinking "herd" mentalities and rethinking the value of the history of public health. *Am J Public Health*. 2023;113(1): 20–21.

Acceptance Date: October 4, 2022.

DOI: https://doi.org/10.2105/AJPH.2022.307148

ACKNOWLEDGMENTS

I wish to thank the editors of *AJPH* for their encouragement and editorial suggestions, and Professor Warwick Anderson for his engagement with the history of epidemiology.

CONFLICTS OF INTEREST

There are no conflicts of interest to report.

REFERENCES

1. Aris Katzourakis, "COVID-19: Endemic Doesn't Mean Harmless," *Nature* 601, no. 7894 (2022): 485, https://doi.org/10.1038/d41586-022-00155-x; Tara Smith, "Will We Ever Get Rid of COVID -19?" *Quanta Magazine*, November 30, 2021; Jacob Steere-Williams, "Endemic Fatalism and Why It Will Not Resolve COVID -19," *Public Health* 206 (February 14, 2022):29–30, https://doi.org/10.1016/j.puhe.2022.02.011; R. U. Mendoza et al., "Public Policy (Not the Coronavirus) Should Shape What Endemic Means," *Journal of Global Health* 12 (2022): 1–5; Scott Knowles and Jacob Steere-Williams, "The Pandemic-Endemic Debate and COVID -19," *COVIDCalls*, February 2, 2022, https://podcasts.apple.com/us/podcast/ep-406-2-2-2022-the-pandemic-endemic-debate-and-covid/id1516341147?i=1000549867791 (accessed October 6, 2022).
2. Warwick Anderson, "The Virus That Therefore I Am," *Science, Technology, & Human Values* (2022): 1–16. https://doi.org/10.1177/01622439221119852
3. Warwick Anderson, "Immunities of the Herd in Peace, War, and COVID-19," *American Journal of Public Health* 112, no. 10 (2022):1465–1470. https://doi.org/10.2105/AJPH.2022.306931
4. Martin Finucane, "Boston Researchers Join Letter in *The Lancet* Rejecting Herd Immunity Strategy," *Boston Globe*, October 14, 2020, cited in Anderson, "Immunities of the Herd in Peace, War, and COVID-19."
5. Olga Amsterdamska, "Demarcating Epidemiology," *Science, Technology, & Human Values* 30, no. 1 (2005): 17–51. https://doi.org/10.1177/0162243904270

Pornography Use and Public Health: Examining the Importance of Online Sexual Behavior in the Health Sciences

Joshua B. Grubbs, PhD, Christopher G. Floyd, MS, and Shane W. Kraus, PhD

ABOUT THE AUTHORS

Joshua B. Grubbs and Christopher G. Floyd are with the Department of Psychology at Bowling Green State University, Bowling Green, OH. Shane W. Kraus is with the Department of Psychology at the University of Nevada Las Vegas.

In 2020, *AJPH* published "Should public health professionals consider pornography a public health crisis?" by Nelson and Rothman.[1] The impetus for this work was clear: in the relatively recent past, 17 states have drafted or passed resolutions calling widespread pornography use a public health crisis, with many US politicians taking the position that pornography use is a threat to public health. The reasons for this contention (i.e., that pornography use is a threat to public health) are varied, though proponents of such a position often contend that pornography is a threat to families, impedes brain development in adolescents, affects brain functioning in adults, is inherently addictive, and promotes a wide variety of illegal sexual activities.[1]

Through their critical review, Nelson and Rothman's work clearly demonstrates that such a position is untenable. Most, if not all, of the contentions made by such legislation and resolutions are entirely unsupported by current research, and pornography use does not meet standard criteria associated with threats to public health (i.e., it is not an acute event requiring immediate response; it does not immediately or directly lead to death, morbidity, or adverse health consequences; it does not overwhelm the capacity of local health care systems).[1] In short, such resolutions are wholly unsupported in both their factual claims and general arguments. Moreover, since 2020, no new states have drafted or passed such resolutions, which may be attributable to the rise of a true public health crisis in 2020.

The impact of Nelson and Rothman's work is both obvious and subtle. Among obvious impacts, their work has been cited widely in a short period of time, generated intense public attention, inspired several op-eds and opinion pieces, and served as a starting point for thousands of conversations via social media (see https://apha.altmetric.com/details/73766659/citations for a summary of the popular media impact of this work). Central to much of this attention has been their conclusion that pornography use is not a public health crisis.

Yet, an equally important implication of the work is overlooked. Nelson and Rothman's work, while showing that pornography is not a public health crisis, demonstrates that pornography use is a topic to be studied by public health. Whereas some disciplines have largely refused to consider pornography use as a topic relevant for inquiry (e.g., *American Psychologist*, the flagship journal of the American Psychological Association, has published nothing on the topic for more than 30 years), public health has engaged with this activity substantively. More directly, Nelson and Rothman demonstrate that seeking to understand pornography use and its effects is a valid domain of inquiry for public health and the health sciences more broadly.

THE SCOPE OF PORNOGRAPHY USE IN THE UNITED STATES

Several recent US nationally representative studies indicate that pornography use is a common recreational activity—equivalent with other digitally mediated behaviors (e.g., video games, social media)—with a majority of men and a sizable plurality of women reporting regular use of pornography.[2–4] Similarly, most US adolescents have seen pornography and indicate that their sexual behaviors may be influenced by pornography exposure and frequency of use.[4]

As previous systematic reviews have shown,[5] there is clear evidence that pornography use, like most sexual behavior, is driven by pleasure-seeking motives. People use pornography to satisfy sexual drive and desire, especially when other sexual options are limited. Not surprisingly, then, for most people, pornography use and concomitant masturbation are normal recreational behaviors that are likely part of a variety of generally healthy sexual behaviors.[5]

The effects of pornography use are mixed.[6] Use is linked to greater sexual objectification of partners, which may be negative in some circumstances.[5] However, it is also associated with greater future openness to and engagement in a range of sexual behaviors and to greater sexual experimentation.[5] In some cases, these links are likely positive (sexual openness being related to greater sexual satisfaction more generally), though there are also associations between pornography use and preferences for or experimentation with more violent and potentially abusive sexual behaviors.[4] Similarly, pornography use is linked to both higher and lower sexual satisfaction,[7] depending on the context of use (dyadic vs solitary).[5] Finally, recent evidence suggests that pornography use is generally unrelated to sexual functioning.[8] More simply, there is very little evidence that pornography use alone inhibits sexual functioning or performance, though this topic remains hotly debated.[8] Collectively then, there is limited evidence that pornography use always or even consistently leads to inherently negative outcomes, but, rather, its effects seem variable depending on a range of individual and sociocultural factors.

Despite the general absence of widespread negative effects stemming from pornography use, such is often encountered in mental health treatment settings.[9] Perhaps the most common reason that practitioners might encounter pornography use as a clinical concern is compulsive use of pornography. Whereas many people use pornography regularly without any reported adverse consequences, there is substantial evidence that pornography use may become out of control, excessive, or impairing for some users.[10] Though there is no psychiatric or mental health diagnosis of "pornography addiction," many people report that they feel as if they cannot control their pornography use or that their pornography use has caused substantial psychosocial functioning impairments.[11]

A recent US national sample found that 10.3% of men and 7% of women at least somewhat agree with the statement "I am addicted to pornography"[12] and that between 25% and 30% of the past-year pornography users reported potential issues in regulating their pornography use.[11] Moreover, the 11th edition of the *International Classification of Diseases* (*ICD-11*) does include a novel diagnosis of compulsive sexual behavior disorder[13] that may subsume compulsive or excessive pornography use, and there is strong reason to suspect that excessive pornography use will be among the most frequent target behaviors associated with the diagnosis.[14] Not surprisingly, then, pornography use is often a reason for individuals seeking treatment, a target behavior for change in psychotherapy and pharmacotherapy interventions, and a commonly encountered issue by mental health practitioners.[9,15,16]

Importantly, there are circumstances wherein pornography use might present as a clinical concern even when it is not deemed excessive or compulsive. For various reasons, people often find the use of pornography to be morally objectionable. However, such condemnation does not always stop people from viewing pornography, and there are now several studies confirming that many people use pornography while still disapproving of it.[17,18] The use of pornography while morally disapproving of pornography gives rise to what past work has labeled moral incongruence. A number of US studies show that, in some circumstances, moral disapproval of pornography amplifies links between use and self-reported addiction,[19] and the use of pornography among those who find it morally wrong is also linked to a greater incidence of depression, lower levels of happiness, lower levels of sexual satisfaction, and greater general distress.[17,18] Ultimately, these effects of moral incongruence have led researchers and clinicians to caution about the importance of accurately assessing the reasons behind someone's decision to seek treatment of problematic pornography use.[14,15]

WHERE DO WE GO FROM HERE?

As Nelson and Rothman's work clearly demonstrates, pornography use is a valid domain of scientific and health-related research. Yet, given the relative novelty of this research domain, particularly in public health and allied fields, there is a need for systematic approaches to understanding this behavior and its effects. Accordingly, here we lay out a series of recommendations for how public health and allied fields might systematically seek to understand pornography use and its effects.

First, we contend that a key aspect to promoting a better understanding of pornography use and its effects is a change in basic assumptions about what behaviors and domains of human functioning are considered rigorous scientific pursuits by the health sciences. Sexual health research has faced stigma in numerous domains,[20] and scientists and health professionals researching such topics are often perceived as unserious or strange.[21,22] Indeed, the recommendations that follow from this point all, in some way or another, presuppose a recognition of research about pornography use and its effects as valid domains of scientific and public health inquiry.

Second, we recommend increased efforts to ensure clinical competence in recognizing, assessing, and treating pornography-related concerns. Such a recommendation is especially salient given the inclusion of compulsive sexual behavior disorder in the *ICD-11*, which may be applied in cases of excessive pornography use.[13] In short, we need better clinical training for mental health clinicians in recognizing both problematic pornography use and normal pornography use. To address this need, national societies and associations, state and regional licensing boards, and specialty organizations are poised to effect immediate change. Among most health and educational professions, continuing education is a mandatory component of ongoing licensure, providing unique and constantly available opportunities to increase clinical competence in these areas.

Given the frequency with which practitioners already encounter pornography use in clinical settings, it is likely that many health professionals already discuss pornography use with their clients. However, as is the case with many sexual behaviors, particularly those that are stigmatized likely because of social mores or traditional sexual values, many clients may feel uncomfortable volunteering information about their pornography use or disclosing sexual preferences. Given such qualms, we recommend that tactful but direct assessments of pornography use be incorporated in normal health screenings as they may provide an opportunity for people to disclose concerns that may have otherwise gone unmentioned. Currently, several measures have been validated in clinical and nonclinical populations, which we have cited throughout this document.[11,14] Akin to alcohol and substance use disorders, routine screening for problematic pornography use would hold many advantages for addressing co-occurring mental health issues among treatment-seeking clients and normalize querying pornography use and other sexual behaviors as a standard part of health care.

Third, we need improved sexual education related to pornography use for both adolescents and the public at large. As previous works have clearly demonstrated, many people use pornography for sexual education purposes.[23] Yet, there is little sexual education material that directly addresses pornography use itself.[24] For many people, particularly adolescents and young adults (aged 18–25 years), it seems that pornography is often functioning as a form of sexual education rather than a topic addressed by comprehensive sexual education. This represents a failing of US sexual education more broadly, as pornography alone is likely not the best or most accurate means of educating oneself about sex or the health risks associated with specific behaviors (e.g., condomless sex). Accordingly, there is a clear need for incorporation of pornography use and pornography-related behaviors into standard, comprehensive sexual education materials during adolescence and in more general sexual health recommendations for the public.

Building on this, given the widespread use of smartphones among US adolescents (95%) and the few safeguards set in place to restrict access to pornography use for adolescents, further work is needed to examine the role of pornography in sexual script formulations on its viewers. Such a need is even more apparent given recent work suggesting that increased pornography consumption is associated with decreased condom use among US adults.[3] Though the links between pornography viewing and condomless sex are less clear in adolescent populations, adolescents are regularly viewing pornography that depicts condomless sex. This speaks to a potential need for limited access to pornography for minors (those younger than 18 years in the United States). One possible means of accomplishing such an aim could be age verification software for pornographic Web sites, like those used in the United States and abroad as a means of restricting access to Web sites that offer gambling, alcohol, and cannabis products.

Fourth, as pornography use is a common and perhaps normal part of modern sexuality, we recommend the consistent integration of pornography use measures into mainstream public health and allied professional research. A simple means of accomplishing this is the regular inclusion of basic questions about the frequency and recency of pornography use in new and ongoing research projects and national surveys for which pornography use might be of relevance. This inclusion of such materials is likely especially relevant for public health research related to sexual behaviors in general, sexual health broadly (including sexually transmitted infections), addictions and addictive behaviors, and relationships. Furthermore, we recommend that researchers begin to use a standardized set of questions when assessing the frequency and recency of pornography use as a means of increasing greater generalizability across studies. An example of such items is available in Appendix A (available as a supplement to the online version of this article at https://ajph.org).

Ultimately, these recommendations demonstrate a need for new funding mechanisms for pornography-related research across disciplines. As previous works have pointed out,[6] it is simply impossible for the scientific and health community to fully understand the effects of pornography without adequate funding. Yet, at present, bills drafted by various states decrying pornography as a public health crisis have not resulted in any substantive funding increases for pornography research. More bluntly, despite widely professed concerns about pornography use, legislatures seem unwilling to put forth the money to support robust research efforts in this domain.

Without established funding priorities for pornography-related research from relatively unbiased agencies, a compromised research agenda could be established, particularly if partisan or ideologically motivated actors were to initiate funding in this domain. The result of biased actors filling the gap left by more traditional scientific funding agencies would likely be a flood of research born from ideology, absent of objectivity and oriented toward predetermined conclusions. Admittedly, pornography use does not currently neatly fit within the research domain criteria for the National Institute of Mental Health, nor does it explicitly comport with the priorities of most US federal funding agencies. Even so, as we have noted throughout this piece, pornography use is clearly salient to public health and allied disciplines, and, thus, it should be funded as such.

CONCLUSIONS

Pornography use is common, and Nelson and Rothman's influential work in *AJPH* clearly demonstrates that, although pornography may not be a public health crisis, this behavior is a salient concern for the field of public health and the health sciences more broadly. All available evidence suggests that pornography is and will continue to be a normal aspect of human sexuality, and, as such, it should be studied rigorously across the behavioral and health sciences.

Based on this, there is a clear and present need for the health sciences and allied professions to

1. designate pornography use an area in need of rigorous academic inquiry;
2. enhance training opportunities for clinicians and professionals who might encounter pornography use in their practice;
3. incorporate pornography use in comprehensive sexual education materials for adolescents and in public health outreach and messaging campaigns around sexual behavior;
4. include questions related to pornography use in ongoing and future research related to sexual behaviors, addiction, sexual health, and relationships; and
5. increase public funding for pornography-related research.

Until these recommendations are met, it is likely that the true public health implications of pornography use will remain poorly understood, despite the clear relevance of the topic to the health sciences. AJPH

CORRESPONDENCE

Correspondence should be sent to Joshua B. Grubbs, Department of Psychology, Bowling Green State University, 822 E Merry Ave, Bowling Green, OH 43403 (e-mail: grubbsj@bgsu.edu). Reprints can be ordered at https://ajph.org by clicking the "Reprints" link.

PUBLICATION INFORMATION

Full Citation: Grubbs JB, Floyd CG, Kraus SW. Pornography use and public health: examining the importance of online sexual behavior in the health sciences. *Am J Public Health*. 2023;113(1):22–26.

Acceptance Date: October 4, 2022.

DOI: https://doi.org/10.2105/AJPH.2022.307146

CONTRIBUTORS

J. B. Grubbs and S. W. Kraus contributed equally to the conceptualization, design, writing, and revisions of this work. C. G. Floyd provided critical revisions. All authors approved the final article.

ACKNOWLEDGMENTS

The authors received no direct funding for this work. J. B. Grubbs and S. W. Kraus receive funding from the Kindbridge Research Institute and the International Center for Responsible Gaming. J. B. Grubbs also receives funding from the Problem Gambling Network of Ohio. S. W. Kraus also receives funding from The Nevada Problem Gambling Project.

The authors would like to thank Kimberly Nelson and Emily Rothman for providing helpful information regarding current legislative processes associated with pornography and public health.

CONFLICTS OF INTEREST

All authors report no conflicts of interest.

REFERENCES

1. Nelson KM, Rothman EF. Should public health professionals consider pornography a public health crisis? *Am J Public Health*. 2020;110(2):151–153. https://doi.org/10.2105/AJPH.2019.305498
2. Regnerus M, Gordon D, Price J. Documenting pornography use in America: a comparative analysis of methodological approaches. *J Sex Res*. 2016; 53(7):873–881. https://doi.org/10.1080/00224499.2015.1096886
3. Wright PJ. Pornography consumption and condomless sex among emerging US adults: results from six nationally representative surveys. *Health Commun*. 2021:1–8. https://doi.org/10.1080/10410236.2021.1917745
4. Herbenick D, Fu TC, Wright P, et al. Diverse sexual behaviors and pornography use: findings from a nationally representative probability survey of Americans aged 18 to 60 years. *J Sex Med*. 2020;17(4):623–633. https://doi.org/10.1016/j.jsxm.2020.01.013
5. Grubbs JB, Wright PJ, Braden AL, Wilt JA, Kraus SW. Internet pornography use and sexual motivation: a systematic review and integration. *Ann Int Commun Assoc*. 2019;43(2):117–155. https://doi.org/10.1080/23808985.2019.1584045
6. Grubbs JB, Kraus SW. Pornography use and psychological science: a call for consideration. *Curr Dir Psychol Sci*. 2021;30(1):68–75. https://doi.org/10.1177/0963721420979594
7. Wright PJ, Tokunaga RS, Kraus A, Klann E. Pornography consumption and satisfaction: a meta-analysis. *Hum Commun Res*. 2017;43(3):315–343. https://doi.org/10.1111/hcre.12108
8. Hoagland KC, Grubbs JB. Pornography use and holistic sexual functioning: a systematic review of recent research. *Curr Addict Rep*. 2021;8(3):408–421. https://doi.org/10.1007/s40429-021-00378-4

9. Short MB, Wetterneck CT, Bistricky SL, Shutter T, Chase TE. Clinicians' beliefs, observations, and treatment effectiveness regarding clients' sexual addiction and internet pornography use. *Community Ment Health J.* 2016;52(8):1070–1081. https://doi.org/10.1007/s10597-016-0034-2
10. Bőthe B, Tóth-Király I, Potenza MN, Orosz G, Demetrovics Z. High-frequency pornography use may not always be problematic. *J Sex Med.* 2020;17(4):793–811. https://doi.org/10.1016/j.jsxm.2020.01.007
11. Kraus SW, Gola M, Grubbs JB, et al. Validation of a brief pornography screen across multiple samples. *J Behav Addict.* 2020;9(2):259–271. https://doi.org/10.1556/2006.2020.00038
12. Grubbs JB, Kraus SW, Perry SL. Self-reported addiction to pornography in a nationally representative sample: the roles of use habits, religiousness, and moral incongruence. *J Behav Addict.* 2019;8(1):88–93. https://doi.org/10.1556/2006.7.2018.134
13. Reed GM, First MB, Billieux J, et al. Emerging experience with selected new categories in the *ICD-11*: complex PTSD, prolonged grief disorder, gaming disorder, and compulsive sexual behaviour disorder. *World Psychiatry.* 2022;21(2):189–213. https://doi.org/10.1002/wps.20960
14. Grubbs JB, Hoagland KC, Lee BN, et al. Sexual addiction 25 years on: a systematic and methodological review of empirical literature and an agenda for future research. *Clin Psychol Rev.* 2020;82:101925. https://doi.org/10.1016/j.cpr.2020.101925
15. Kraus SW, Sweeney PJ. Hitting the target: considerations for differential diagnosis when treating individuals for problematic use of pornography. *Arch Sex Behav.* 2019;48(2):431–435. https://doi.org/10.1007/s10508-018-1301-9
16. Lew-Starowicz M, Draps M, Kowalewska E, Kraus SW, Gola M. Tolerability and efficacy of paroxetine and naltrexone for treatment of compulsive sexual behaviour disorder. *World Psychiatry.* 2022;21(3):468–469. https://doi.org/10.1002/wps.21026
17. Grubbs JB, Perry SL, Wilt JA, Reid RC. Pornography problems due to moral incongruence: an integrative model with a systematic review and meta-analysis. *Arch Sex Behav.* 2019;48(2):397–415. https://doi.org/10.1007/s10508-018-1248-x
18. Floyd CG, Grubbs JB. Context matters: how religion and morality shape pornography use Effects. *Curr Sex Health Rep.* 2022;14(3):82–98. https://doi.org/10.1007/s11930-022-00329-8
19. Grubbs JB, Kraus SW, Perry SL, Lewczuk K, Gola M. Moral incongruence and compulsive sexual behavior: results from cross-sectional interactions and parallel growth curve analyses. *J Abnorm Psychol.* 2020;129(3):266–278. https://doi.org/10.1037/abn0000501
20. Irvine JM. Is sexuality research 'dirty work'? Institutionalized stigma in the production of sexual knowledge. *Sexualities.* 2014;17(5-6):632–656. https://doi.org/10.1177/1363460713516338
21. Msibi T. Contextualising 'dirty work': a response to Janice Irvine (2014). *Sexualities.* 2014;17(5–6):669–673. https://doi.org/10.1177/1363460714531278
22. Štulhofer A. Reflections from the periphery: a commentary on Irvine. *Sexualities.* 2014;17(5–6):681–685. https://doi.org/10.1177/1363460714531275
23. Rothman EF, Beckmeyer JJ, Herbenick D, Fu TC, Dodge B, Fortenberry JD. The prevalence of using pornography for information about how to have sex: findings from a nationally representative survey of US adolescents and young adults. *Arch Sex Behav.* 2021;50(2):629–646. https://doi.org/10.1007/s10508-020-01877-7
24. Rothman EF, Adhia A, Christensen TT, Paruk J, Alder J, Daley N. A pornography literacy class for youth: results of a feasibility and efficacy pilot study. *Am J Sex Educ.* 2018;13(1):1–17. https://doi.org/10.1080/15546128.2018.1437100

Cigarette Use Among Older Adults: A Forgotten Population

Bethea A. Kleykamp, PhD, MA, and Jessica A. Kulak, PhD, MPH, MS

ABOUT THE AUTHORS

Bethea A. Kleykamp is owner and principal of BAK and Associates, Baltimore, MD. Jessica A. Kulak is with the Department of Community Health and Health Behavior, School of Public Health and Health Professions, University at Buffalo, Buffalo, NY.

The number of adults aged 65 years and older is expected to more than double worldwide over the next several decades, and for the first time in recorded history, older adults will outnumber children (https://bit.ly/3D4p0im). Despite these unprecedented population shifts, older adults are significantly underrepresented in biomedical research, especially in the field of nicotine and tobacco science (https://bit.ly/3shUSuI). This focus on younger cohorts has obscured the reality that combustible tobacco use (i.e., smoking) has remained virtually unchanged for older adults for nearly two decades in the United States (Figure 1).

Meanwhile, smoking prevalences among youths and young adults in the United States are at the lowest levels ever recorded. One explanation for these differences in prevalence trajectories could be that, since at least 2005, quit rates among older smokers have remained stagnant (https://bit.ly/3NaxXeF).[1] Aligning with this observation is evidence suggesting that traditional tobacco control policies (i.e., pricing, smoke-free policies, information campaigns, bans on advertising, health warning labels, cessation treatments) are not affecting older smokers the same as younger cohorts, as represented in an analysis of smoking behavior in Europe between 2004 and 2013 (https://bit.ly/3VVs2y2). Additionally, older smokers may have less knowledge of quitlines or other local smoking cessation services[2,3] and more misconceptions about the relative harms of nicotine and combustible tobacco.[2] Older adults are also less likely to use noncombustible nicotine products (https://bit.ly/3z3iZAY).

The lack of attention paid to older smokers does not match the incredible burden of disease and death that this population carries. Tobacco-related disease is age-related disease as evidenced by older smokers incurring 12 times greater health care expenses than middle-aged smokers (https://bit.ly/3eXhLR8).[4] As noted by the American Cancer Society, cancers associated with smoking are most often diagnosed after the age of 65 years and include lung, kidney, bladder, and stomach cancer (https://bit.ly/3F7gtxB). Although most people start smoking in the early part of their life, most suffering and deaths associated with tobacco use occur far later. Unfortunately, older adult smokers are not represented in the most basic methodological details of nicotine and tobacco research. For example, in other fields of study, "older adults" are often defined as those who are 65 years and older and may be further delineated as the young old (65–74 years), middle old (75–84 years), and old old (≥ 85 years).[5] However, research on tobacco use does not adhere to this definition, with studies defining "older adults" across a wide range of ages (e.g., 25 years or older; https://bit.ly/3TljwAr). Beyond this, many studies explicitly exclude anyone older than 65 years from participation (https://bit.ly/3VP032T). These inconsistencies in definitions and study inclusion criteria can confound what we know about tobacco use among older adults.

Adding to these disparities is the reality that older smokers face a range of socially and medically complex challenges. In the United States, older smokers are more likely to be American Indian/Alaska Native, Black, or multiracial; to have less than a high school education; and to earn less than $25 000 a year (https://bit.ly/3TpJzfP). The intersection of age and race is notable, particularly when examining smoking cessation behaviors. Older Black men are less likely to stop smoking as they age than are older White men despite starting smoking later in life.[6] Older Black smokers are also disproportionately excluded from lung cancer screening guidelines despite this population facing a higher risk of lung cancer.[7] Older adults in the United States are less likely to use the Internet for health-related information seeking,[8] which may heighten inequalities in health information access. Compounding these health equity issues are the multitude of comorbid health conditions associated with tobacco smoking, that could increase the likelihood of age-related psychosocial and physical

AJPH January 2023, Vol 113, No. 1

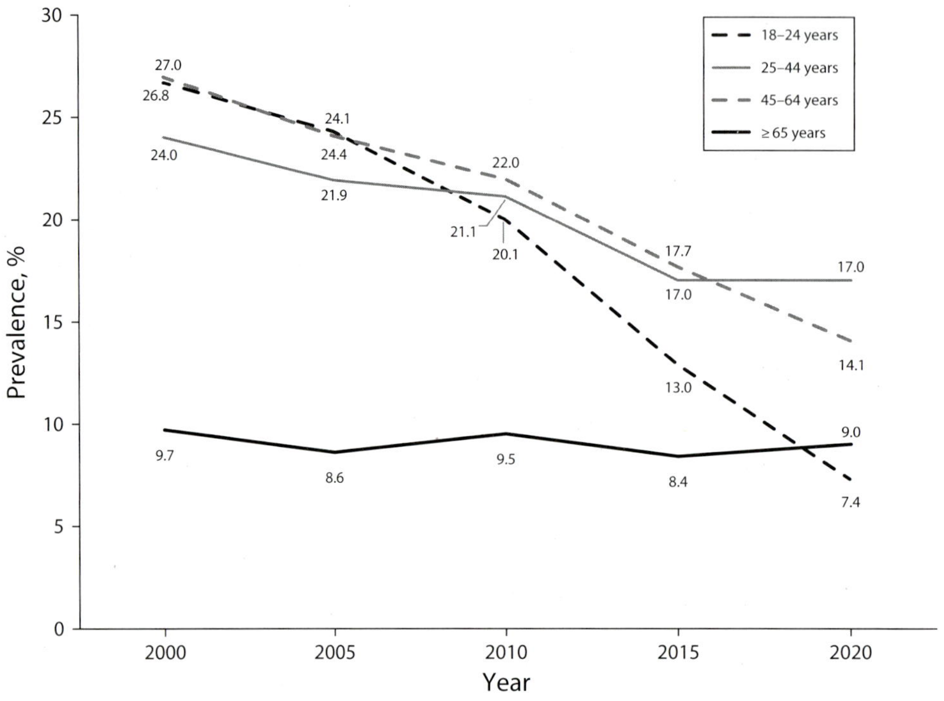

FIGURE 1— Current Cigarette Smoking Among Adults Aged 18 Years and Older, by Age: United States, 2000–2020

Note. The National Health Interview Survey (NHIS) defines current cigarette smokers, represented in the figure, as those who had smoked 100 or more cigarettes in their lifetime and, at the time of the interview, smoked every day or some days.
Source. Data are from the NHIS and are published in *Morbidity and Mortality Weekly Reports* for each year represented (https://bit.ly/3MT3nWE).

health conditions such as chronic pain, dementia, and social isolation or loneliness.

One rarely discussed option for addressing the health of aging smokers is harm reduction. The topic of tobacco harm reduction has become a lightning rod for disagreement because of ongoing concerns that novel nicotine products such as electronic cigarettes (e-cigarettes) could damage the health of nonsmokers, including youths. Although efforts to prevent the uptake of tobacco and nicotine use among young people are critical, they should not supersede a focus on the lives of older smokers. Prioritizing dependence prevention over harm reduction is not ethically justified.[9] Like harm reduction approaches for other substance use disorders and geriatric patients facing chronic health conditions, such as obesity, tobacco harm reduction philosophy respects the autonomy and health goals of older adults who might be ambiguous about smoking cessation. Such smokers could benefit from learning that reducing the number of cigarettes smoked can significantly lower their mortality risk (https://bit.ly/3guzMqj) or that the predominant cause of cancer is combustible tobacco, not nicotine.

Although previous research indicates that the public largely does not have a good understanding of harm reduction as it relates to nicotine products (https://bit.ly/3TH4MSV), emerging ethical frameworks cautiously support the adoption of noncombustible nicotine products, such as electronic cigarettes, as a harm reduction alternative to smoking.[10] Clinicians working with older adults should consider emphasizing the differential risks associated with smoking compared with noncombustible products (https://bit.ly/3Sr6KFe). Messages can support the cessation of all nicotine and tobacco products while simultaneously providing education about differential product risk and adhering to principles of informed consent and consumer autonomy (https://bit.ly/3Sr6KFe). Furthermore, clinicians working with older adults may wish to develop graphical risk messaging, as people are more likely to accurately perceive tobacco product risk and to share that information with others when risk messaging is graphics-based as opposed to text-based (https://bit.ly/3f2pqgS).

Future work should explore whether this type of risk messaging is effective for older adult smokers. Likewise, clinicians and others providing cessation support to older adults should tailor their messaging to this population, with attention to acknowledging behavioral stage, beliefs about the harms of smoking and benefits of quitting, supporting motivation and self-efficacy, and ensuring adequate and timely social support.[11] Clinicians and research teams should be reminded that older adult smokers want to quit smoking and can still experience benefits from cessation (https://bit.ly/3TOgEIl).[11,12]

Efforts to rectify the age-related disparities we have described are imperative and must include strategic approaches for educating and motivating older smokers to reduce or stop their use of smoked tobacco. Older adults are not a homogenous group, and intervention efforts must consider social and environmental factors contributing to their health behaviors. Unfortunately, funding opportunities and public health interventions are rarely tailored to older adults, leaving a significant gap in what we understand about the older smoker's experience or what interventions best help older adults. Key research gaps include the degree of nicotine dependence among older smokers and its relationship with quitting smoking. In addition, operational definitions used to define smoking history such as the 30 or more pack-years used in lung cancer screening eligibility[7] should be evaluated to better understand whether such definitions are perpetuating health inequalities among Black and other minority older adult smokers. Finally, understanding the efficacy and effectiveness of noncombustible nicotine products, such as e-cigarettes, and how they might aid older adults' smoking cessation attempts is warranted. Certainly, there are challenges to adopting a harm reduction framework, and continued surveillance of the long-term effects of e-cigarettes and other noncombustible tobacco products among older adults is needed.

Older smokers deserve to know that it is never too late to improve their health and that quitting smoking can add years to their lives regardless of age (https://bit.ly/3guzMqj). Future research efforts focused on developing novel, age-tailored interventions are critical for public health, including efforts to address smoking among older people historically marginalized because of age, race, education level, and income. Otherwise, the status quo will continue, and the suffering and early death of millions of older adult smokers will persist. AJPH

CORRESPONDENCE

Correspondence should be sent to Bethea (Annie) Kleykamp, MA, PhD, BAK and Associates, LLC, 906 S Clinton St, Baltimore, MD 21224 (e-mail: akleykamp@gmail.com). Reprints can be ordered at http://www.ajph.org by clicking the "Reprints" link.

PUBLICATION INFORMATION

Full Citation: Kleykamp BA, Kulak JA. Cigarette use among older adults: a forgotten population. *Am J Public Health*. 2023;113(1):27–29.

Acceptance Date: October 10, 2022.

DOI: https://doi.org/10.2105/AJPH.2022.307151

CONTRIBUTORS

B. A. Kleykamp wrote the first draft of the editorial. Both authors revised and finalized the editorial.

CONFLICTS OF INTEREST

During the past 36 months, B. A. Kleykamp has received compensation for full-time work from the US Food and Drug Administration–supported public–private partnership ACTTION (https://www.acttion.org) and the American Society of Addiction Medicine (ASAM). B. A. Kleykamp is also the owner of BAK and Associates, a research consulting and science writing firm. Contracts include work for nonprofits, ASAM, the ECRI Institute, the health technology assessment company Hayes, Inc./Symplr, the real-world evidence company STATinMED, the government contractor Palladian Associates, and the health care consulting company PinneyAssociates. The work for PinneyAssociates was completed in 2021 and focused on regulatory submissions related to psychedelic drugs. None of this work was funded by the nicotine or tobacco industries. B. A. Kleykamp has also received honorarium payments totaling US $700 for articles published in Filter (https://filtermag.org/about-the-influence-foundation) and PBS Next Avenue (https://www.nextavenue.org/about-us). J. A. Kulak has no conflicts of interest to declare.

REFERENCES

1. Isenberg JY, Quiñones AR, Slatore CG, Bryson WC, Thielke SM. Trends in cigarette smoking and cessation among Medicare managed care recipients, 2005–2012. *Addict Behav*. 2016;58:155–160. https://doi.org/10.1016/j.addbeh.2016.02.037
2. Kulak JA, LaValley S. Cigarette use and smoking beliefs among older Americans: findings from a nationally representative survey. *J Addict Dis*. 2018;37(1–2):46–54. https://doi.org/10.1080/10550887.2018.1521255
3. Kerr S, Watson H, Tolson D, Lough M, Brown M. Smoking after the age of 65 years: a qualitative exploration of older current and former smokers' views on smoking, stopping smoking, and smoking cessation resources and services. *Health Soc Care Community*. 2006;14(6):572–582. https://doi.org/10.1111/j.1365-2524.2006.00659.x
4. Maciosek MV, Xu X, Butani AL, Pechacek TF. Smoking-attributable medical expenditures by age, sex, and smoking status estimated using a relative risk approach. *Prev Med*. 2015;77:162–167. https://doi.org/10.1016/j.ypmed.2015.05.019
5. Sharma M, Branscum PW. *Introduction to Community and Public Health*. 2nd ed. Hoboken, NJ: Wiley; 2020.
6. Holford TR, Levy DT, Meza R. Comparison of smoking history patterns among African American and White cohorts in the United States born 1890 to 1990. *Nicotine Tob Res*. 2016;18(suppl 1):S16–S29. https://doi.org/10.1093/ntr/ntv274
7. Li CC, Matthews AK, Rywant MM, Hallgren E, Shah RC. Racial disparities in eligibility for low-dose computed tomography lung cancer screening among older adults with a history of smoking. *Cancer Causes Control*. 2019;30(3):235–240. https://doi.org/10.1007/s10552-018-1092-2
8. Jacobs W, Amuta AO, Jeon KC. Health information seeking in the digital age: An analysis of health information seeking behavior among US adults. *Cogent Soc Sci*. 2017;3(1):1302785. https://doi.org/10.1080/23311886.2017.1302785
9. Magalhaes M. Vaping restrictions: is priority to the young justified? *Nicotine Tob Res*. 2021;23(1):32–35. https://doi.org/10.1093/ntr/ntaa175
10. Franck C, Filion KB, Kimmelman J, Grad R, Eisenberg MJ. Ethical considerations of e-cigarette use for tobacco harm reduction. *Respir Res*. 2016;17(1):53. https://doi.org/10.1186/s12931-016-0370-3
11. Rimer BK, Orleans CT, Fleisher L, et al. Does tailoring matter? The impact of a tailored guide on ratings and short-term smoking-related outcomes for older smokers. *Health Educ Res*. 1994;9(1):69–84. https://doi.org/10.1093/her/9.1.69
12. Avila JC, Berg CJ, Robinson J, Ahluwalia JS. Short and long-term cigarette and tobacco abstinence among daily and non-daily older smokers. *Nicotine Tob Res*. 2022; Epub ahead of print. https://doi.org/10.1093/ntr/ntac116.

Social Disparities in the Duration of Power and Piped Water Outages in Texas After Winter Storm Uri

Sara E. Grineski, PhD, Timothy W. Collins, PhD, Jayajit Chakraborty, PhD, Eric Goodwin, MS, Jacob Aun, MA, and Kevin D. Ramos

We assessed sociodemographic disparities in basic service disruptions caused by Winter Storm Uri in Texas. We collected data through a bilingual telephone survey conducted in July 2021 (n = 753). Being Black, having children, and renting one's residence were associated with longer power outage durations; being Black was also associated with longer water outages. Our findings highlight the need to plan for and ameliorate inequitable service outages and their attendant health risks in climate change–related extreme weather events such as Uri. (*Am J Public Health*. 2023;113(1):30–34. https://doi.org/10.2105/AJPH.2022.307110)

AJPH January 2023, Vol 113, No. 1

Winter Storm "Uri" included three arctic fronts that swept across the state of Texas from February 10 through 20, 2021. Treating Uri as a natural intervention, we examine sociodemographic disparities in power and water outage durations associated with the storm.

INTERVENTION AND IMPLEMENTATION

We treat Uri as a natural intervention because it triggered major societal disruptions. As numerous counties faced extreme low temperatures, 10 million people lost access to electricity[1] because electricity and gas systems were insufficiently winterized, the major electric grid operator (i.e., Electric Reliability Council of Texas) was isolated from the national grid and unable to import power, and some power plants were out of service for planned maintenance.[2] One study inferred that 69% of Texans went without power and 49% went without running water.[3] Power outage conditions directly caused 210 deaths (e.g., from carbon monoxide poisoning); when indirect causes are included, Uri led to an estimated 700 deaths.[2] Texas incurred $130 billion in economic losses as a result of the storm.[1] To understand the unequal effects of this event, we conducted a 35-minute telephone survey in English and Spanish across eight Texas metropolitan statistical areas in July 2021.

PLACE, TIME, AND PERSONS

The survey was administered to randomly selected residents 18 years or older in counties representing the following Texas metropolitan statistical areas: Dallas–Fort Worth, Houston, San Antonio, Austin, McAllen, El Paso, Beaumont–Port Arthur, and Lubbock (Figure A, available as a supplement to the online version of this article at http://www.ajph.org). The sampling frame was proportionally weighted according to the population (n = 1964). Of 1764 eligible respondents contacted, 896 (50.8%) completed the survey. We excluded 143 respondents who did not complete survey items used to construct three or more of our analysis variables, leaving a final sample size of 753.

We collected data on sociodemographic characteristics (independent variables) and the durations of power and water outages (in hours) associated with the storm, the latter two of which we analyzed as dependent variables. Descriptive statistics for all variables are shown in Table 1. To analyze the data, we used multiple imputation to address missing values and then employed our multiply imputed data in multivariable generalized estimating equation models.

PURPOSE

It is important to study events such as Uri because they cause power[4,5] and

TABLE 1— Descriptive Statistics Pertaining to a Household Survey Conducted in Eight Texas Metropolitan Statistical Areas: 2021

Variable	No. Households	Minimum	Maximum	Mean ±SD	Yes, No. (%)	No, No. (%)	Missing, (%)
Total hours home was without electricity	745	0.0	504.0	42.156 ±55.914			1.0
Total hours home was without piped water service	724	0.0	672.0	32.691 ±68.762			4.0
Household income[a]	734	1	10	5.260 ±2.868			0.3
Householder race/ethnicity							
Non-Hispanic White	748	0	1		329 (44.0)	419 (56.0)	0.7
Non-Hispanic Black	748	0	1		81 (10.8)	667 (89.2)	0.7
Hispanic	752	0	1		265 (35.2)	487 (64.8)	0.1
Non-Hispanic other	748	0	1		71 (9.5)	677 (90.5)	0.7
US-born householder	746	0	1		616 (82.6)	130 (17.4)	0.9
Household has a disabled member	753	0	1		341 (45.3)	412 (54.7)	0.0
Household has a member older than 65 y	743	0	1		271 (36.5)	472 (63.5)	1.3
Household has a child (or children)	750	0	1		289 (38.5)	461 (61.5)	0.4
Ownership status							
Owns	753	0	1		497 (66.0)	256 (34.0)	0.0
Rents, non-HUD	753	0	1		133 (17.7)	620 (82.3)	0.0
Rents from HUD	753	0	1		123 (16.3)	630 (83.7)	0.0
ERCOT power grid[b]	753	0	1		667 (88.6)	86 (11.4)	0.0
Freeze severity[c]	753	1.53	23.15	15.028 ±4.030			0.0

Note. ERCOT = Electric Reliability Council of Texas; HUD = Housing and Urban Development. The household sample size was 753.

[a]Income variable categories were as follows: (1) < $10 000, (2) $10 000–$19 999, (3) $20 000–$29 999, (4) $30 000–$39 999, (5) $40 000–$49 999, (6) $50 000–$74 999, (7) $75 000–$99 999, (8) $100 000–$149 999, (9) $150 000–$249 999, and (10) ≥ $250 000.

[b]Data were not collected via our survey; we used Geographic Information System software to overlay geocoded locations of our respondents (based on household addresses) with a power grid polygon shapefile.

[c]Data were not collected via our survey; we used secondary data to create this measure. Freeze severity is a measure of the extent to which the minimum temperature during the storm deviated from the average minimum temperature. We calculated the minimum temperature that occurred between February 10 and 20, 2021, for each household on the basis of High-Resolution Rapid Refresh radar data. We then subtracted the average February minimum temperature in each metropolitan statistical area.

water[6,7] outages, which pose serious risks to public health. Disasters tend to disproportionately affect socially disadvantaged communities that lack resources to stay safe and recover quickly.[8] Because of the lack of outage data, few published studies have examined inequities in power and water outages. During Uri, an ecological analysis revealed that Texas counties with more severe power outages had greater concentrations of Hispanic residents.[2] A report on an Internet survey conducted after Uri showed minimal differences in reported outage durations between racial/ethnic groups[3] but lacked statistical testing and examination of other covariates. Another report showed that one tenth of the population in predominantly White areas suffered a nighttime blackout during Uri, as compared with one half in areas with large concentrations of racial/ethnic minority residents.[9]

Our survey data provide a unique basis for statistically examining household-level inequalities in the self-reported durations of both power and water outages during Uri. We addressed the following question: How were sociodemographic characteristics associated with the duration of basic service outages during Uri across the eight Texas metropolitan areas assessed?

EVALUATION AND ADVERSE EFFECTS

Observed means for power and water loss durations were 42 hours and 33 hours, respectively. In the multivariable generalized estimating equation models, being Black, having children, and renting one's residence were associated with longer power outages; being Black was associated with longer water outages (all *P*s < .05; Table 2). To determine how much longer, we used the

TABLE 2— Pooled Results of Multivariable Generalized Estimating Equations Including Data Collected Through a Household Survey Conducted in Eight Texas Metropolitan Statistical Areas: 2021

	Duration of Power Outage, b (95% CI)	Duration of Piped Water Outage, b (95% CI)
Intercept	2.76 (1.74, 3.79)	25.80 (4.80, 46.81)
2020 household income	−0.01 (−0.04, 0.03)	−1.62 (−3.49, 0.24)
Householder race/ethnicity		
Non-Hispanic White	0 (Ref)	0 (Ref)
Non-Hispanic Black	0.52 (0.30, 0.75)	25.34 (5.40, 45.33)
Hispanic	0.12 (−0.098, 0.34)	6.03 (−3.94, 16.01)
Non-Hispanic other	0.02 (−0.13, 0.30)	−0.57 (−15.08, 13.93)
Householder country of origin		
Foreign-born	0 (Ref)	0 (Ref)
US-born	0.14 (−0.14, 0.41)	−1.99 (−14.07, 10.09)
Household composition		
All household members are younger than 65 y	0 (Ref)	0 (Ref)
Household has an older member	0.05 (−0.17, 0.27)	0.56 (−10.49, 11.62)
Household has a disabled member	0.02 (−0.13, 0.16)	2.25 (−7.09, 11.59)
Household has a child (or children)	0.35 (0.19, 0.52)	5.20 (−5.64, 16.04)
Ownership status		
Owns	0 (Ref)	0 (Ref)
Rents, non-HUD	0.44 (0.12, 0.76)	12.85 (−2.20, 27.91)
Rents from HUD	0.14 (−0.08, 0.36)	13.72 (−3.60, 30.97)
ERCOT power grid	0.33 (−0.69, 1.34)	6.94 (−21.53, 35.41)
Freeze severity	0.03 (−0.01, 0.08)	1.07 (−1.03, 3.16)

Note. CI = confidence interval; ERCOT = Electric Reliability Council of Texas; HUD = Housing and Urban Development. The household sample size was 753. The term pooled results refers to our use of multiple imputation to address missing values. We created 20 data sets with separate imputed values for missing observations and used these data in our pooled statistical analyses. Model specifications are normal with log link (for duration of power outage) and normal with identity link (for duration of piped water outage), with an exchangeable correlation matrix and clustering of metropolitan statistical areas (n = 8) by median age of housing stock categories (n = 8). Models also controlled for five winter climatic zone categories on the basis of average annual minimum winter temperature. Parameter estimate sizes are not comparable between the models owing to different model specifications (i.e., link functions). Collinearity diagnostics indicated an absence of multicollinearity in these models. SPSS version 28.0 (IBM, Somers, NY) was used in generating our models.

models in Table 2 to calculate estimated marginal means. In contrast to observed means (Table 1), estimated marginal means adjust for covariates (i.e., all other variables held at their observed means) and multivariable model specifications (Table 2). The model for power outage duration predicted 58.6 hours versus 34.8 hours for Black versus non-Hispanic White householders, 45.7 hours versus 34.3 hours for households with children versus those without, and 41.4 hours versus 32.1 hours for renters versus owners. For water outage duration, the model predicted 57.0 hours versus 31.6 hours for Black versus non-Hispanic White householders.

These significant findings were robust according to sensitivity analyses of multiply imputed data for all cases (n = 896; Table A, available as a supplement to the online version of this article at http://www.ajph.org), cases with complete data only (n = 699; Table B, available as a supplement to the online version of this article at http://www.ajph.org), and cases without outlier dependent variable values (n = 746 and n = 743; Table C, available as a supplement to the online version of this article at http://www.ajph.org). The only exceptions, when comparing the sensitivity analyses to the Table 2 findings, were the renter status–longer power outage finding becoming statistically nonsignificant (Tables B and C); Electric Reliability Council of Texas grid, public housing residence, and being US born becoming statistically significant for longer power outages (Table C); and renter status becoming statistically significant for longer water outages (Table C).

In terms of limitations, survey data were collected five months after the event, which could have led to recall bias. We do not know whether there was nonresponse bias in the sample. In addition, we did not model locations of critical facilities, the presence of which reduced the chance of blackouts by approximately 6% during Uri.[9]

SUSTAINABILITY

Research on social disparities associated with events such as Uri is important and should be prioritized. Because of climate change[10] and the public health effects of service outages,[4–7] Uri should serve as a bellwether nationwide. Black householders, householders with children, and renters experienced disproportionately longer outages and should be targeted with public health interventions, including provision of bottled water, small grants to purchase food, and blankets and warm jackets (especially when cold weather occurs in warm climates[11]). At a societal level, improving infrastructure systems to withstand extreme weather and equitably protect residents is of utmost public health importance.

PUBLIC HEALTH SIGNIFICANCE

Whereas previous research has highlighted disparities in power outages in minority areas[9] and Hispanic areas[2] in Texas during Uri, we found power outages of significantly longer durations for Black households. Households with children and renters also reported longer power outages. During a winter storm, power outages lead to relatively cold indoor temperatures, and cold is a leading cause of mortality; the attributable mortality rate in the United States for cold temperatures is an order of magnitude larger than it is for high temperatures.[12] Long-duration power and water outages are stressful for households as toilets cannot be flushed and lights cannot be turned on; furthermore, there are substantial economic costs associated with replacing food and buying bottled water. These stressors disproportionately affected Black householders, householders with children, and renters after Uri.

Gastrointestinal issues are a health risk associated with basic service outages. Black households likely faced increased risks of gastrointestinal issues after Uri because of their longer power and water outage durations relative to White households. One study showed that adolescents and adults with diarrhea after a daylong power outage in New York City were more than 2.5 times as likely as those without diarrhea to have consumed seafood and meats.[4] Although the Centers for Disease Control and Prevention recommends avoiding refrigerated food once power outages exceed four hours, that time window stretches to 24 to 48 hours for half-full and full freezers. Black households' outages exceeded the 48-hour window during which food would still edible, whereas White households' outages did not.

In addition, a systematic review revealed that gastrointestinal issues are associated with longer versus shorter water outages because pipes become increasingly vulnerable to backflow and intrusion.[6] This implies that Black households likely faced higher risks of gastrointestinal issues than White households after Uri because of the disproportionately longer outages they endured. AJPH

ABOUT THE AUTHORS

Sara E. Grineski is with the Department of Sociology, University of Utah, Salt Lake City. Timothy W. Collins, Eric Goodwin, and Kevin D. Ramos are with the Department of Geography, University of Utah. Jayajit Chakraborty and Jacob Aun are with the Department of Sociology and Anthropology, University of Texas at El Paso.

CORRESPONDENCE

Correspondence should be sent to Sara E. Grineski, University of Utah Department of Sociology, 380 S 1530 E Room 301, Salt Lake City, UT 84112 (e-mail: sara.grineski@soc.utah.edu). Reprints can be ordered at http://www.ajph.org by clicking the "Reprints" link.

PUBLICATION INFORMATION

Full Citation: Grineski SE, Collins TW, Chakraborty J, Goodwin E, Aun J, Ramos KD. Social disparities in the duration of power and piped water outages in Texas after Winter Storm Uri. *Am J Public Health*. 2023;113(1):30–34.

Acceptance Date: August 29, 2022.

DOI: https://doi.org/10.2105/AJPH.2022.307110

CONTRIBUTORS

S. E. Grineski conceptualized and conducted the statistical analysis and wrote the first draft of the article. T. W. Collins and J. Chakraborty advised on the study design and statistical analysis and contributed to the writing of the article. E. Goodwin, J. Aun, and K. D. Ramos prepared the non-survey-based data for the project and contributed to the writing of the article. S. E. Grineski, T. W. Collins, and J. Chakraborty obtained the funding for the project.

ACKNOWLEDGMENTS

This article is based on work supported by the National Science Foundation under grants CMMI-2127941 and CMMI-2127932, and the National Institute of Environmental Health Sciences under award R25 ES031497.

We gratefully acknowledge the survey participants for taking the time to be part of our study.

CONFLICTS OF INTEREST

The authors report no conflicts of interest.

HUMAN PARTICIPANT PROTECTION

This project was declared exempt by the institutional review boards of the University of Utah and the University of Texas at El Paso as per exemption category 2.

REFERENCES

1. Busby JW, Baker K, Bazilian MD, et al. Cascading risks: understanding the 2021 winter blackout in Texas. *Energy Res Soc Sci*. 2021;77:102106. https://doi.org/10.1016/j.erss.2021.102106
2. Flores NM, McBrien H, Do V, Kiang MV, Schlegelmilch J, Casey JA. The 2021 Texas power crisis: distribution, duration, and disparities. *J Expo Sci Environ Epidemiol*. 2022 [Epub ahead of print]. https://doi.org/10.1038/s41370-022-00462-5

3. Watson K, Crock R, Jones M. The winter storm of 2021. Available at: https://uh.edu/hobby/winter 2021/storm.pdf. Accessed April 14, 2022.
4. Marx MA, Rodriguez CV, Greenko J, et al. Diarrheal illness detected through syndromic surveillance after a massive power outage: New York City, August 2003. *Am J Public Health.* 2006;96(3): 547–553. https://doi.org/10.2105/AJPH.2004.061358
5. Casey JA, Fukurai M, Hernández D, Balsari S, Kiang MV. Power outages and community health: a narrative review. *Curr Environ Health Rep.* 2020; 7(4):371–383. https://doi.org/10.1007/s40572-020-00295-0
6. Ercumen A, Gruber JS, Colford JMJ. Water distribution system deficiencies and gastrointestinal illness: a systematic review and meta-analysis. *Environ Health Perspect.* 2014;122(7):651–660. https://doi.org/10.1289/ehp.1306912
7. Säve-Söderbergh M, Bylund J, Malm A, Simonsson M, Toljander J. Gastrointestinal illness linked to incidents in drinking water distribution networks in Sweden. *Water Res.* 2017;122:503–511. https://doi.org/10.1016/j.watres.2017.06.013
8. Wisner B, Blaikie P, Cannon T, Davis I. *At Risk: Natural Hazards, People's Vulnerability and Disasters.* 2nd ed. London, England: Routledge; 2004.
9. Carvallo J, Chi Hsu F, Shah Z, Jay T. Frozen out in Texas: blackouts and inequity. Available at: https://www.rockefellerfoundation.org/case-study/frozen-out-in-texas-blackouts-and-inequity. Accessed June 29, 2022.
10. National Academies of Sciences, Engineering, and Medicine. Attribution of extreme weather events in the context of climate change. Available at: https://nap.nationalacademies.org/catalog/21852/attribution-of-extreme-weather-events-in-the-context-of-climate-change. Accessed July 1, 2022.
11. Li D, Zhang Y, Li X, Meyer M, Bazan M, Brown R. "I didn't know what to expect or what to do": impacts of a severe winter storm on residents of subsidized housing in Texas. Available at: https://ssrn.com/abstract=4047541. Accessed June 29, 2022.
12. Burkart KG, Brauer M, Aravkin AY, et al. Estimating the cause-specific relative risks of non-optimal temperature on daily mortality: a two-part modelling approach applied to the Global Burden of Disease Study. *Lancet.* 2021;398(10301):685–697. https://doi.org/10.1016/S0140-6736(21)01700-1

Embracing Advanced Methodology to Improve Population Health

Roger Vaughan, DrPH, MS

ABOUT THE AUTHOR

Roger Vaughan is an associate editor for AJPH *and is with the Department of Biostatistics at The Rockefeller University Hospital, New York, NY.*

See also Seewald, p. 37, Bauer et al., p. 40, Wang and Chakraborty, p. 49, and Liu et al., p. 60.

AJPH has long endorsed the application of novel and powerful state-of-the-art methodological approaches to advance population health. In 2004, we asked David Murray[1,2] and Allan Donner,[3] two pioneers in the development and application of group or cluster randomized trials, to provide extensive primers on their design, application, and analysis, and invited them to help keep these tools in our analytic toolbox by providing methodological updates in 2017.[4,5]

In 2018, we embraced the notion of returning "cause" to our public health vocabulary, and employing causal inference methods to our data when appropriate. Miguel Hernan[6] and others[7] presented a compelling case that while, for many good historical reasons, we kept our expectation of finding and stating causes to a minimum and similarly kept our language away from the term, that it was time to acknowledge that we are indeed after causes. And while we may not be in a design or analytic space to suggest cause, we should not shy away from the application of methods for causal inference when appropriate and should strive to push our research as far down the causal pathway as possible. In 2023, *AJPH* is again promoting the adoption of advanced methodologies to improve population health with the presentation of three methodologies and approaches.

METHODOLOGICAL ADVANCES

First, Wang and Chakraborty (p. 49) present an outstanding review of a method that overcomes some of the downsides of traditional randomized controlled trials, which often tend to compare one novel treatment to standard or usual care, where participants remain in their assigned treatment groups over the life of the trial. Such trials can often last months or years and can be prohibitively expensive. The sequential multiple assignment randomized trial (SMART) and other such adaptive or dynamic treatment strategies allow investigators to reassign patients to additional intervention arms depending upon response to the previous intervention. The review paper offers an overview of methods and applications and provides links to R code and methods for sample size calculations for SMARTs as well as for the statistical analysis of such trials. A supportive commentary by Seewald in this issue also extends the conversation and provides further insights into the application of SMART designs (Seewald p. 37).

Second, Liu et al. (p. 60) expertly present the design and analysis considerations for a whole class of interventions that recognize that spatially and temporally static interventions are not always optimal. These "just-in-time adaptive interventions" (JITAIs) seek to provide the most effective intervention type at just the right time and place; in a smoking cessation program, a JITAI approach might send reminders to a participant to check their patch or chew replacement therapy gum during periods of high craving, while sending alerts to practice meditation, to exercise, or participate in healthy and alternative behaviors during other times, and perhaps deliver no intervention when all internal and external conditions are optimal for cessation so as not to overburden the patient. Liu et al. describe a design approach, microrandomized trials (MRTs), that are employed to help determine the type and duration of those spatially and temporally optimal interventions. Liu et al. use two published examples of the implementation and analysis of MRTs and provide tables with comprehensive links to published methods and R, SAS, or Stata code for both sample size calculations for, and statistical analysis of, MRTs, whose results can be used to populate the content of JITAIs.

Third, Bauer et al. (p. 40) describe a Bayesian estimation method to help identify testing disparities and inform the magnitude of testing deficiency in the context of small area estimation, using severe acute respiratory syndrome coronavirus 2 (SARS-CoV-2) as an example. Bauer et al. present a two-step sampling method that has a number of advantages over traditional approaches. First, just as "all politics are local," all public health is local as well, and the method is designed to be implemented in smaller, local environments where testing data and information may be sparse.

Second, it can help, in real time, predict the number of tests that will be needed to better inform the supply chain needs and can incorporate the often-dynamic parameters of a pandemic rather than relying on fixed and perhaps outdated inputs. In a public health catch-22, areas with fewer available tests may report lower rates, thereby reinforcing the false need for fewer tests. As in the article by Hernan,[7] in which he observes that the terror evoked by the term "causal inference" may keep many away from implementing causal methods, uttering the word "Bayesian" may similarly keep investigators at bay. Fortunately, Bauer et al. (p.40) provide links to the necessary R code on GitHub along with a practice data set for easy implementation.

PUSH–PULL

Methodologies and population health often operate in a symbiotic push–pull relationship, in which stubborn health issues push the development of novel design and analytic methodologies, and new methodologies allow for interrogations to get pulled into new areas and offer potential solutions. We hope that by presenting these methods in user-friendly formats that it makes it easier to enter the population health push–pull conversation and continue to advance health. AJPH

CORRESPONDENCE

Correspondence should be sent to Roger Vaughan, MS, DrPH, The Rockefeller University, 1230 York Ave, New York, NY 10065 (e-mail: roger.vaughan@rockefeller.edu). Reprints can be ordered at https://ajph.org by clicking the "Reprints" link.

PUBLICATION INFORMATION

Full Citation: Vaughan R. Embracing advanced methodology to improve population health. *Am J Public Health*. 2023;113(1):35–36.

Acceptance Date: October 19, 2022.

DOI: https://ajph.org/10.2105/AJPH.2022.307155

CONFLICTS OF INTEREST

The author has no conflicts of interest to declare.

REFERENCES

1. Murray DM, Varnell SP, Blitstein JL. Design and analysis of group-randomized trials: a review of recent methodological developments. *Am J Public Health*. 2004;94(3):423–432. https://doi.org/10.2105/AJPH.94.3.423
2. Varnell SP, Murray DM, Janega JB, Blitstein JL. Design and analysis of group-randomized trials: a review of recent practices. *Am J Public Health*. 2004;94(3):393–399. https://doi.org/10.2105/ajph.94.3.393
3. Donner A, Klar N. Pitfalls of and controversies in cluster randomization trials. *Am J Public Health*. 2004;94(3):416–422. https://doi.org/10.2105/AJPH.94.3.416
4. Turner EL, Li F, Gallis JA, Prague M, Murray DM. Review of recent methodological developments in group-randomized trials: part 1—design. *Am J Public Health*. 2017;107(6):907–915. https://doi.org/10.2105/AJPH.2017.303706
5. Turner EL, Prague M, Gallis JA, Li F, Murray DM. Review of recent methodological developments in group-randomized trials: part 2—analysis. *Am J Public Health*. 2017;107(7):1078–1086. https://doi.org/10.2105/AJPH.2017.303707
6. Hernán MA. The C-word: scientific euphemisms do not improve causal inference from observational data. *Am J Public Health*. 2018;108(5):616–619. https://doi.org/10.2105/AJPH.2018.304337
7. Galea S, Vaughan RD. Moving beyond the cause constraint: a public health of consequence, May 2018. *Am J Public Health*. 2018;108(5):602–603. https://doi.org/10.2105/AJPH.2018.304390

Adaptive Interventions for a Dynamic and Responsive Public Health Approach

Nicholas J. Seewald, PhD

ABOUT THE AUTHOR

Nicholas J. Seewald is with the Department of Health Policy and Management, Johns Hopkins Bloomberg School of Public Health, Baltimore, MD.

See also Vaughan, p. 35, Bauer et al., p. 40, Wang and Chakraborty, p. 49, and Liu et al., p. 60.

Wang and Chakraborty's article in this issue of *AJPH* (p. 49) provides a fantastic summary of developments in the design and analysis of sequential, multiple-assignment randomized trials (SMARTs), alongside examples in which these trials can be used to improve infectious disease control. Sequentially randomized trials are powerful tools for developing evidence-based interventions that can adapt to individuals' changing needs over time. In this comment, I focus on adaptive interventions themselves, separated from a study design, to advocate for their increased development and dissemination not only in infectious disease research, but in public health more broadly.

Fundamentally, SMARTs are tools that allow for the development of high-quality adaptive interventions (also commonly called dynamic treatment regimens or adaptive treatment strategies). Adaptive interventions are sequences of decision rules that map ongoing information about individuals, clinics, geographical areas, or other types of treated units onto recommendations for subsequent treatment.[1] In this way, adaptive interventions operationalize real-life clinical and public health practice. High-quality adaptive interventions provide principled guidance on how to modify an intervention when and for whom it is necessary. Critically, an adaptive intervention is a fixed sequence of recommendations that guide treatment decisions: it is an *intervention* design, whereas a SMART is a *study* design that can answer questions about the development of adaptive interventions.

Questions about how to construct an effective adaptive intervention take many forms. They can be as simple as, "How should we initiate treatment to maximize effectiveness?", "How should we modify treatment for units for which the initial intervention does not work?", or "Should we provide a maintenance intervention for those units that responded well to the initial treatment, or just watch and wait?" Other questions might be about how to identify individuals or units whose first-stage treatment should be modified, or how long one should wait before treatment modification. Fundamentally, these are questions about bundling interventions in sequences that recognize and leverage treatment effect heterogeneity to achieve better public health outcomes.[2]

In the malaria SMART discussed by Wang and Chakraborty, the investigators recognize that the dynamic nature of malaria risk, along with rising insecticide resistance, necessitates adaptation: single interventions or standard combinations thereof may not be enough to control malaria in Africa.[3] In this context and many others, treatments that work in one region or for one group of individuals may not work for another, and treatments that work now may not work in the future. This is widely acknowledged, but there is still a dearth of research examining the effects of interventions working in concert with one another—as they do in practice—rather than as stand-alone, one-size-fits-all approaches to treatment.[2] Additionally, the adaptive interventions embedded in this SMART consider cost-effectiveness by reserving expensive interventions like larval source management for those sites where low-cost interventions were insufficient for reducing malaria incidence.

The American Public Health Association believes that equity is at the core of public health.[4] Adaptive interventions are of interest not only because they mimic actual public health practice, but also because they can help improve outcomes for everyone. By explicitly recommending intervention strategies for both responders and nonresponders, adaptive interventions provide a principled "backup plan" for those for whom the initial intervention is insufficient. In the COVID-19 example SMART described by Wang and Chakraborty, the trial design explicitly studies ways to motivate those individuals still unvaccinated after initial outreach.[5] If the trial discovers an effective adaptive intervention, it will be one that has

AJPH January 2023, Vol 113, No. 1

considered the needs of those non-responding individuals. Single-stage interventions cannot do this.

SMARTs are a powerful tool for addressing open questions about multiple stages of an adaptive intervention. But, as Wang and Chakraborty point out, they are not the only randomized trial design that facilitates research on adaptive interventions.[6] SMARTs are a means to an end: they exist to enable research into questions about adaptive interventions. As with any study design, those scientific questions must come first, and a SMART should only be designed if justified by the science. In some cases, the scientific questions may require a different, possibly simpler, trial design.[7] Additionally, randomization is not always feasible or ethical, in which case a randomized trial cannot be used at all.

In a rapidly evolving infectious disease context, such as the early COVID-19 pandemic, nonexperimental methods for identifying effective treatments and prevention strategies can be crucial. Just as there is a growing literature on methods for constructing adaptive interventions from SMARTs, similar innovation is happening in nonexperimental settings. Through the use of hospital records or data from an epidemiological surveillance system, for example, statistical reinforcement learning methods can be used to discover effective adaptive interventions.[8] These methods rely on natural variation in treatment provision over time to identify adaptive interventions that optimize the outcome of interest, and use causal inference techniques to avoid bias due to confounding.[9] Although SMARTs and other randomized trials remain the gold standard, other approaches to research on adaptive interventions do exist and can be used when randomization is difficult or impossible.

Wang and Chakraborty rightly point out the need for methodological innovations that improve the speed and efficiency of SMARTs. These methods will be critical for the design's adoption in time-sensitive scenarios like evolving epidemics or pandemics. Cluster-randomized SMARTs are likely to be an important tool in developing adaptive interventions for infectious disease control and prevention, just as cluster-randomized single-stage trials are. Adaptive randomization and interim monitoring techniques can help as well by allowing principled on-the-fly changes to the design that increase the number of participants receiving treatment recommendations from an effective adaptive intervention. Bringing in other methods from the singly randomized trial literature, such as covariate adjustment and early stopping procedures, may also help improve the efficiency of SMARTs.

Although development of adaptive interventions has been of growing interest, there remains a sizeable gap between research and practice. SMARTs are frequently described as optimization trials, not confirmatory ones. Indeed, Murphy's seminal 2005 article on SMARTs explicitly says that these trials should be viewed as part of a series of developmental studies leading to a confirmatory trial.[10] To the best of my knowledge, adaptive interventions informed by SMARTs are rarely if ever tested against standard of care in a confirmatory trial, even nearly 20 years after the design's introduction. Suitable control groups can and have been built into SMARTs by embedding one adaptive intervention that recommends standard of care throughout, but rarely are these trials powered for comparisons of other embedded adaptive interventions against that control. Methods for powering trials for identifying an optimal adaptive intervention exist, but translational work is required to make them accessible to nonstatisticians.[11] Additionally, more attention should be paid to rolling out and scaling up high-quality, evidence-based adaptive interventions; advances in implementation science to support putting these multistage, tailored interventions into practice are needed.

Wang and Chakraborty provide a thorough introduction to SMARTs and their possible use in infectious disease research. Adaptive interventions have the potential to improve outcomes across fields by emphasizing combinations of effective treatments delivered sequentially when and to whom they are needed. Although methodological and implementation challenges remain, adaptive interventions can be powerful, cost-effective tools to promote public health. Wang and Chakraborty have developed an excellent resource for scholars looking to develop adaptive interventions to bring us toward a more dynamic, responsive vision for public health. AJPH

CORRESPONDENCE

Correspondence should be sent to Nicholas J. Seewald, 624 N. Broadway, Room 501, Baltimore, MD 21205 (e-mail: nseewal1@jhu.edu). Reprints can be ordered at http://www.ajph.org by clicking the "Reprints" link.

PUBLICATION INFORMATION

Full Citation: Seewald NJ. Adaptive interventions for a dynamic and responsive public health approach. *Am J Public Health.* 2023;113(1):37–39.

Acceptance Date: October 17, 2022.

DOI: https://doi.org/10.2105/AJPH.2022.307157

ACKNOWLEDGMENTS

Research reported in this publication was supported by the National Institute of Mental Health of the National Institutes of Health (award no. P50MH115842).

Note. The contents are solely the responsibility of the author and do not necessarily represent the official views of the National Institutes of Health.

CONFLICTS OF INTEREST

The author has no conflicts of interest to declare.

REFERENCES

1. Collins LM, Murphy SA, Bierman KL. A Conceptual framework for adaptive preventive interventions. *Prev Sci.* 2004;5(3):185–196. https://doi.org/10.1023/B:PREV.0000037641.26017.00
2. Lei H, Nahum-Shani I, Lynch K, Oslin D, Murphy SAA. "SMART" design for building individualized treatment sequences. *Annu Rev Clin Psychol.* 2012;8(1):21–48. https://doi.org/10.1146/annurev-clinpsy-032511-143152
3. Zhou G, Lee M, Atieli HE, et al. Adaptive interventions for optimizing malaria control: an implementation study protocol for a block-cluster randomized, sequential multiple assignment trial. *Trials.* 2020;21(1):665. https://doi.org/10.1186/s13063-020-04573-y
4. American Public Health Association. 10 essential public health services. Available at: https://www.apha.org/What-is-Public-Health/10-Essential-Public-Health-Services. Accessed October 11, 2022.
5. Dai H, Saccardo S, Han MA, et al. Behavioural nudges increase COVID-19 vaccinations. *Nature.* 2021;597(7876):404–409. https://doi.org/10.1038/s41586-021-03843-2
6. Almirall D, Nahum-Shani I, Wang L, Kasari C. Experimental designs for research on adaptive interventions: singly and sequentially randomized trials. In: Collins LM, Kugler KC, eds. *Optimization of Behavioral, Biobehavioral, and Biomedical Interventions: Advanced Topics.* Statistics for Social and Behavioral Sciences. Cham, Switzerland: Springer International Publishing; 2018:89–120. https://doi.org/10.1007/978-3-319-91776-4_4
7. Nahum-Shani I, Dziak JJ, Wetter DW. MCMTC: a pragmatic framework for selecting an experimental design to inform the development of digital interventions. *Frontiers in Digital Health.* 2022. Available at: https://www.frontiersin.org/articles/10.3389/fdgth.2022.798025. Accessed October 12, 2022.
8. Chakraborty B, Moodie EEM. *Statistical Methods for Dynamic Treatment Regimes.* New York, NY: Springer New York; 2013. https://doi.org/10.1007/978-1-4614-7428-9
9. Mahar RK, McGuinness MB, Chakraborty B, Carlin JB, IJzerman MJ, Simpson JA. A scoping review of studies using observational data to optimise dynamic treatment regimens. *BMC Med Res Methodol.* 2021;21(1):21–39. https://doi.org/10.1186/s12874-021-01211-2
10. Murphy SA. An experimental design for the development of adaptive treatment strategies. *Stat Med.* 2005;24(10):1455–1481. https://doi.org/10.1002/sim.2022
11. Rose EJ, Laber EB, Davidian M, Tsiatis AA, Zhao YQ, Kosorok MR. Sample size calculations for SMARTs. *arXiv:190606646 [stat].* June 2019. Available at: http://arxiv.org/abs/1906.06646. Accessed July 9, 2019.

A Novel Bayesian Spatial–Temporal Approach to Quantify SARS-CoV-2 Testing Disparities for Small Area Estimation

Cici Bauer, PhD, Xiaona Li, MPH, Kehe Zhang, MS, Miryoung Lee, PhD, Esmeralda Guajardo, MA, Susan Fisher-Hoch, MD, Joseph McCormick, MD, Maria E. Fernandez, PhD, and Belinda Reininger, DrPH

See also Vaughan, p. 35, Seewald, p. 37, Wang and Chakraborty, p. 49, and Liu et al., p. 60.

Objectives. To propose a novel Bayesian spatial–temporal approach to identify and quantify severe acute respiratory syndrome coronavirus 2 (SARS-CoV-2) testing disparities for small area estimation.

Methods. In step 1, we used a Bayesian inseparable space–time model framework to estimate the testing positivity rate (TPR) at geographically granular areas of the census block groups (CBGs). In step 2, we adopted a rank-based approach to compare the estimated TPR and the testing rate to identify areas with testing deficiency and quantify the number of needed tests. We used weekly SARS-CoV-2 infection and testing surveillance data from Cameron County, Texas, between March 2020 and February 2022 to demonstrate the usefulness of our proposed approach.

Results. We identified the CBGs that had experienced substantial testing deficiency, quantified the number of tests that should have been conducted in these areas, and evaluated the short- and long-term testing disparities.

Conclusions. Our proposed analytical framework offers policymakers and public health practitioners a tool for understanding SARS-CoV-2 testing disparities in geographically small communities. It could also aid COVID-19 response planning and inform intervention programs to improve goal setting and strategy implementation in SARS-CoV-2 testing uptake. (*Am J Public Health*. 2023;113(1):40–48. https://doi.org/10.2105/AJPH.2022.307127)

Since the COVID-19 pandemic started, a growing body of literature has revealed disparities in severe acute respiratory syndrome coronavirus 2 (SARS-CoV-2) testing. For example, minority communities of Blacks and Hispanics had lower testing rates.[1] Language barriers and lack of health insurance have also been identified as barriers to SARS-CoV-2 testing.[2,3] Geographical disparities in SARS-CoV-2 testing have been recognized in many studies.[4,5] SARS-CoV-2 testing rates were lower in rural states and higher in well-off suburbs with predominantly White populations.[6,7] Most studies have adopted an ecological analysis of SARS-CoV-2 testing in US counties to examine testing disparities geographically and the association between testing and various area-level contextual factors. Although many found evidence of testing disparities, they rarely quantified the testing gap; in other words, they rarely answered the question: How many tests should be done to remove the disparity?

One exception is Dryden-Peterson et al.,[8] who proposed a rank-based approach to quantify the number of tests needed by zip code tabulation areas in Massachusetts to bridge the disparities in SARS-CoV-2 testing. This approach makes minimal assumptions about data distribution and other factors contributing to testing and infection patterns (e.g., vaccination and nonpharmaceutical interventions). Moreover, ranks are performed to compare areas relative to each other in the study region, so this approach could be more informative to local public health departments for planning and resource allocation.

AJPH January 2023, Vol 113, No. 1

Although such a rank-based approach is appealing, some issues are also noted, particularly in the context of small area estimation.[9] First, when the geographic areas are small or the relevant population is small, the observed test positivity rate (TPR)—usually calculated as the ratio of the number of positive cases to the number of tests conducted on a daily or weekly basis—would be highly variable and often as extreme as 0% or 100%. In some situations, such as when there are zero tests performed in a specific area or time frame, it is impossible to accurately estimate the number of positive infections (e.g., TPR would be 0/0 mathematically). Second, from a practical perspective, the rank-based approach to examining testing disparity would be more useful if the assessment could be made prospectively, as opposed to retrospectively. For example, if the testing gap (by rate or by number) could be quantified for the weeks ahead, it could greatly support local health departments and health practitioners in setting goals for resource allocation, community outreach and engagement, and educational programs.

The National Institutes of Health–funded Rapid Acceleration of Diagnostics–Underserved Populations (RADx–UP) projects, which focus on enhancing SARS-CoV-2 testing among health disparate populations, could also benefit from the quantification of testing gaps. Indeed, our motivation for developing the proposed 2-step Bayesian spatial–temporal approach arose from the gaps and limitations related to small geographical areas experienced by authors and key community stakeholders in their practice and research responses to the COVID-19 pandemic.

We illustrate the rank-based algorithm proposed by Dryden-Peterson et al.[8] in detail and demonstrate the issues of directly applying this approach for small area estimation. We apply our approach to SARS-CoV-2 testing and infection surveillance data from Cameron County, Texas, where over 90% of the population is Mexican American.[10] Cameron County is also one of the study sites of an ongoing RADx–UP project.[11]

METHODS

We illustrate the issues of the existing rank-based algorithm in small area estimation and describe our proposed Bayesian spatial–temporal approach.

Rank-Based Approach

To illustrate the algorithm proposed by Dryden-Peterson et al.,[8] we used mock data from Table 1 and adapted values from the actual Cameron County COVID-19 surveillance database between March 2020 and February 2022. Let m_{it} denote the number of SARS-CoV-2 tests reported in area (e.g., zip code tabulation areas) i ($i=1, \cdots, I$) at time point t ($t=1, \cdots, T$), and y_{it} denote the number of detected positive cases. To assess the testing disparity, we needed measures of the testing intensity r_{it} (representing the supply aspect) and the epidemic intensity p_{it} (representing the demand aspect). The observed testing intensity was quantified as the testing rate per 10 000 population, calculated as $\hat{r}_{it} = \left(\frac{m_{it}}{N_{it}}\right) \times 10\,000$, with N_{it} being the population size.

The epidemic intensity is measured by the TPR, calculated as $\hat{p}_{it} = y_{it}/m_{it}$ using the observed testing and case numbers. For a given time point t, we ranked areas in the study region by the testing intensity $\hat{r}_{it}$ (e.g., from the lowest to the highest)

TABLE 1— Mock Data Illustrating the Rank-Based Approach to Assessing the Testing Gap Proposed in Dryden-Peterson et al.[8]

GEOID	Population, No.	Testing Frequency	Testing Rate per 10 000	Rank of Testing Rate	Positive Frequency	TPR	Rank of TPR	Gap Exists?	Testing Gaps, No.
GEO1	1190	20	168.1	5	2	0.10	1	No	0
GEO2	1095	10	91.3	2	2	0.20	2	No	0
GEO3	1000	10	100.0	3	5	0.50	4	Yes	4
GEO4	1200	16	133.3	4	4	0.25	3	No	0
GEO5	880	1	11.4	1	1	1.00	5	Yes	14
GEO6	1790	0	0.0	...	0	0	...	...	...

Note. GEOID = geographic ID; TPR = test positivity rate. Testing frequency was the number of tests performed for a given area and time. We calculated TPR as the ratio of the number of cases to the number of tests performed. Positive frequency was the number of tested positive cases for a given area and time. We adopted values in the table from the Cameron County COVID-19 surveillance data between March 2020 and February 2022, with the actual GEOID masked and population size slightly adjusted for privacy purposes. GEO6 presented the case this algorithm could not handle and motivated the Bayesian 2-step approach we propose.

and by the epidemic intensity $\hat{p}_{it}$. Our rationale for the rank-based comparison was that if the supply met the demand, the rank of the supply would match the rank of the demand; otherwise, the rank of the supply would be lower than the rank of the demand. In the context of SARS-CoV-2 testing disparities, an area would be considered to have a testing deficiency if its rank of epidemic intensity (i.e., $\hat{p}_{it}$) was higher than its rank of test intensity (i.e., $\hat{r}_{it}$). We calculated the number of tests needed to remove the deficiency as the additional number of tests required to achieve the matching ranks after accounting for the different population sizes by area.

The algorithm can be seen more clearly using the data in Table 1. We present SARS-CoV-2 testing and case data from 6 census block groups (CBGs) in Cameron County. The observed testing frequency ranged from 0 to 20, and the number of positive cases ranged from 0 to 5. We first calculated the test intensity rates (we used per 10 000 population because the CBG-level population size was small) and the TPRs. For example, for area GEO1, the test intensity rate was 168.1 (calculated as [20/1190] × 10 000), and TPR was 0.1 (2/20). At first, we considered only the areas GEO1–GEO5 because GEO6 presented a special issue that we will describe later.

We ranked the 5 areas respective to the testing rate and TPR from lowest to highest. For area GEO1, because its rank of testing rate (i.e., fifth) was higher than its rank of TPR (i.e., first), there was no testing deficiency. For area GEO5, its rank of testing rate (i.e., first) was lower than that of its TPR (i.e., fifth), and hence there was a testing deficiency. To calculate the needed tests, one would first locate the area with the testing rate rank matching the corresponding TPR. For GEO5 with TPR ranking fifth, we located the area with the testing rate ranking fifth—GEO1—because the testing rate for GEO1 was 168.1 per 10 000 population and so should be the expected testing rate for GEO5. After accounting for the population size in GEO5, the expected test frequency was 168.1 × 880/10 000 = 14.8. The difference between the expected and the observed test frequency was then 14.8 − 1 = 13.8, or 14 tests, rounding up. Therefore, there were testing disparities in GEO5, and 14 additional tests should have been performed to address the deficiency.

Although easily implemented by software such as Excel, this algorithm fails to accommodate the case of GEO6, as it has zero tests and zero cases. On one hand, one may argue that zero cases suggest no expected infection, and hence there was no testing deficiency for this area. On the other hand, one could argue that areas with zero tests indicate the highest testing deficiency and hence should be prioritized for testing. Moreover, for area GEO5, the observed TPR of 100% lacks accuracy because of the small number of tests performed (i.e., 1). These issues motivated our proposed Bayesian 2-step approach.

Proposed Bayesian 2-Step Approach

The 2-step approach we propose addressed the estimation and prediction of testing disparity in the context of small area estimation. It has broader applications beyond COVID-19 testing and could be used as a routine analytical framework for infectious disease surveillance systems.

Proposed 2-step approach. In step 1, we employed the Bayesian inseparable space–time models originally proposed in Knorr-Held,[12] which has been popular in disease-mapping models,[13] including models of COVID-19 outcomes.[14] These models provided the estimated TPR, denoted by p_{it} for area i and time t, with accuracy for small area estimation improved by borrowing information across time and space.[15,16] We assumed the observed number of positive cases Y_{it} to follow a binomial distribution with the parameter p_{it}:

$$(1) \qquad Y_{it} \sim Binom(m_{it},\, p_{it}),$$

where m_{it} denoted the total tests performed in area i and time t. On the logit scale, we decomposed the positive rate p_{it} additively as

$$(2) \qquad \text{logit}(p_{it}) = \mu + \mathbf{X}_{it}\boldsymbol{\beta} + u_i + v_i + \psi_t + \gamma_t + \delta_{it}.$$

Here, $\mathbf{X}_{it}$ denotes a vector of potential risk factors or barriers for area i at time t, which could include area-level characteristics, such as the percentage of the population without health insurance, or the percentage of the population vaccinated—if such data were available. The parameter vector $\exp(\boldsymbol{\beta})$ estimated the odds ratio of infection associated with those risk factors. The main spatial effect was modeled as the Besag-York-Mollié model,[17] with a structured spatial component $\mathbf{u}$ and an unstructured spatial component $\mathbf{v}$. We assumed the structured component to have an intrinsic conditional autoregressive model and the unstructured component to have a normal distribution $N_I(0, \sigma_v^2\mathbf{I})$, where $\mathbf{I}$ indicates the identity matrix, and σ_v^2 the corresponding variance parameter.

We modeled the main temporal effect additively with a structured temporal effect $\boldsymbol{\psi}$ and an unstructured temporal effect $\boldsymbol{\gamma}$, assuming $\boldsymbol{\psi}$ to have a second-order random walk (to impose temporal smoothing) and $\boldsymbol{\gamma}$ to have a normal distribution: $N_T(0, \sigma_\gamma^2\mathbf{I})$. The space–time interaction term $\boldsymbol{\delta}$ can take 4 different forms as the product of 1 of the spatial main effects (i.e., **u** and **v**) and 1 of the temporal main effects (i.e., $\boldsymbol{\psi}$ and $\boldsymbol{\gamma}$). More details of the model specification can be found in the supplementary materials (available as a supplement to the online version of this article at http://www.ajph.org). We used a conditional predictive ordinate for model selection.[18] Our main interest was the estimated p_{it} but not the individual spatial or temporal component. The inseparable model provided the smoothing needed for the observed TPR with an extreme value (e.g., 100%); moreover, it allowed our imputation of the TPR for areas with 0 tests performed (i.e., $m_{it}=0$). This can be done by setting the observed Y_{it} to NA and the corresponding m_{it} to 1 when fitting the model. We chose the noninformative priors used previously.[12] We used the posterior mean and the 95% credible intervals (95% CrI) when making our inference of the estimated TPR.

In step 2, we ranked the areas using the estimated TPRs from step 1 and then assessed the testing deficiency and calculated the additionally needed tests in the same way as the rank-based approach.

Prospectively predicting the testing gap using the proposed 2-step approach for testing planning. The Bayesian inseparable space–time models allow short-term prediction of the TPR for future events. We emphasize that the prediction is regarding future events and should not be confused with the fitted values from statistical modeling, which are often called the "predicted values." For example, Lieberman-Cribbin et al.[19] used "prediction" to present the estimated positivity rate from fitting a Poisson regression model, which differed from the prediction we are proposing. The predicted TPRs, denoted by $\tilde{p}_{i,t+1}$ or $\tilde{p}_{i,t+2}$, would be obtained from the Bayesian model in step 1. The testing deficiency would be performed by comparing the ranks using predicted TPRs to the ranks of testing intensity at current time t. Other ways to quantify the infection intensity instead of the TPR, such as case acceleration rates or the "doubling rate" of cases for the past weeks, can also be used in ranking.

We assessed the testing gap in 3 ways, reflecting the immediate, short-term, and long-term disparities. We tested the immediate testing disparity by comparing the predicted TPR $\tilde{p}_{i,t+1}$ at week $t+1$ to the current testing rate $\hat{r}_{it}$ at week t. The rank difference between these 2 rates would give the expected tests and hence the testing deficiency. Because the testing rate often fluctuated every week, we compared the predicted TPR to the average testing rate from the previous month for the short-term testing disparity. Finally, we compared the predicted TPR to the average testing rate across the entire study window (i.e., from the time the pandemic started to the time of analysis) for ranking to obtain the long-term testing disparity.

We implemented the proposed method in R version 3.6.3 and R package INLA (R Foundation for Statistical Computing, Vienna, Austria).[20] R code to implement the proposed approach is available at http://bit.ly/3UPLmLI, along with a simulated data set.

RESULTS

We have demonstrated our proposed 2-step approach to SARS-CoV-2 testing disparities in Cameron County, Texas. Cameron County is located in the Lower Rio Grande Valley in south Texas on the US–Mexico border and is among the poorest of US counties, with more than 30% of its residents living in poverty.[10] The prevalence of several chronic disease conditions that have been identified as comorbidities that increase the risk of COVID-19 infection and severity is also exceptionally high, with type 2 diabetes more than 27% and obesity more than 50%.[21–23] More than 90% of the population is Mexican American,[10] and similar to other minority groups, this population has seen disproportionately high infection and fatality rates since the first local reported cases of COVID-19 on March 18, 2020.

Several COVID-19 mitigation responses led by local public health departments and government–academic partnerships for community-based intervention programs have focused on improving SARS-CoV-2 testing and vaccination in Cameron County. The mitigation strategies targeted small, defined areas of the county where populations with health disparities (e.g., low income, low educational attainment, crowding) reside. When conducting education and outreach (particularly door-to-door) efforts, information about the testing pattern at granular spatial levels such as the CBGs is more desirable. The CBG-level population size was approximately 1900 on average and ranged from 208 to 14 481; the small population size posed special challenges to providing accurate estimates of infection and testing.

A total of 667 052 SARS-CoV-2 testing records were reported in Cameron County between March 18, 2020 and February 10, 2022. Of these, 70 795 (10.6%) were positive. We were able to geocode the majority (89.9%) of the testing records to obtain the corresponding CBG. We included only the polymerase chain reaction (PCR) tests (71.7% of all reported tests) in quantifying the testing gap because SAR-CoV-2 infection was confirmed only by the

PCR test. We included 222 CBGs in our analysis (shown in Section A, available as a supplement to the online version of this article at http://www.ajph.org, for the geography). The data-processing flowchart is presented in Section B (available as a supplement to the online version of this article at http://www.ajph.org). The weekly trend of SARS-CoV-2 infection and testing patterns for Cameron County as a whole had 4 distinctive peaks (shown in Section C, available as a supplement to the online version of this article at http://www.ajph.org). However, we observed substantial variation in both infection and testing rates at the CBG level.

We applied our proposed approach to weekly CBG-level testing data. Based on the conditional predictive ordinate, we considered the Bayesian inseparable model with type II interaction the best, so we used it for inference. Detailed results from all models can be found in Sections E through G (available as a supplement to the online version of this article at http://www.ajph.org). Figure 1 presents the temporal trends of the observed TPRs (black dots) and model-based TPRs (blue line, with 95% CrIs in a lighter shade) from 6 selected CBGs. Areas 1 and 2 represent CBGs with relatively large population sizes (~14 000 and ~13 000, respectively; we do not include the exact population size to avoid identification of specific areas), and the TPRs were fairly stable and followed the overall pattern at the county level. Areas 3 through 6 represented CBGs with much smaller population sizes: from approximately 300 to approximately 1000 individuals. Given the sparse testing data, the observed TPRs fluctuated substantially from week to week, with many extreme values of 0% and 100%. Moreover, these areas also had weeks when no tests were conducted; hence there is no observed TPR (dots not shown).

Our model fitted the observed data very well: for areas with sufficient tests (areas 1 and 2), the fitted lines followed the observed points very closely. For areas with sparse tests (areas 4–6), model-based estimates provided the needed shrinkage on extreme values of the observed TPR, which better reflected the underlying infection trend. Meanwhile, although the model borrowed information across CBGs, it also preserved any local pattern that deviated from the overall county trend (e.g., in area 3). After we obtained the model-based TPR, we calculated the testing deficiency by week for each CBG. Figure 2 presents the number of additional tests needed during the study time frame, in which the county-level TPR was overlaid (red line) with the y-axis scale on the right. Figure 2, panel a, displays the number of CBGs (of the total 222) that we identified as having a testing gap, and panel b presents the variation of additional tests from these CBGs. Throughout the period, 217 of the 222 CBGs experienced testing deficiency at some point. The testing deficiency ranged substantially and differed by waves. Our analysis also suggested that substantial tests should have been performed even during the low infection period (e.g., February–May 2021).

Figure 3 presents the predicted testing disparity by CBG based on the predicted TPR for the week of February 7, 2022, using all observed data from March 18, 2020 through February 7, 2022. For the immediate testing disparity, we used the testing rate from the preceding week (i.e., January 31–February 6, 2022) for testing ranks. For short- and long-term disparities, we used the testing rate from the preceding month (i.e., January 10–February 6, 2022) and the average testing rate across the entire study period (i.e., March 18, 2020–February 6, 2022), respectively. Although the areas with immediate or short-term testing deficiencies tended to have increased infection rates, the areas predicted to have long-term testing disparity tended to be more rural and experienced limited access to care (including COVID-19 testing) even before the COVID-19 pandemic.

DISCUSSION

We have demonstrated our proposed novel Bayesian 2-step approach to identifying SARS-CoV-2 testing disparities and quantifying testing deficiencies in the context of small area estimation. Our analytical framework can provide key information to aid local public health departments in COVID-19 response planning and inform intervention programs, such as RADx-UP, to improve goal setting and strategic implementation of interventions to increase SARS-CoV-2 testing uptake.

Strengths

Our proposed analysis has several advantages over those proposed in other studies for identifying SARS-CoV-2 testing disparities. First, we developed a novel statistical framework and a data-driven approach to understanding testing disparity in the context of small area estimation. To our knowledge, this is the first study to evaluate population-level SARS-CoV-2 testing deficiencies with the spatial granularity of CBGs. Second, we provided a sophisticated spatial–temporal approach to better estimate infection intensity (e.g., TPRs) with sparse or no testing data, so that one can assess testing disparities more accurately. Third, we went beyond the qualitative assessment of

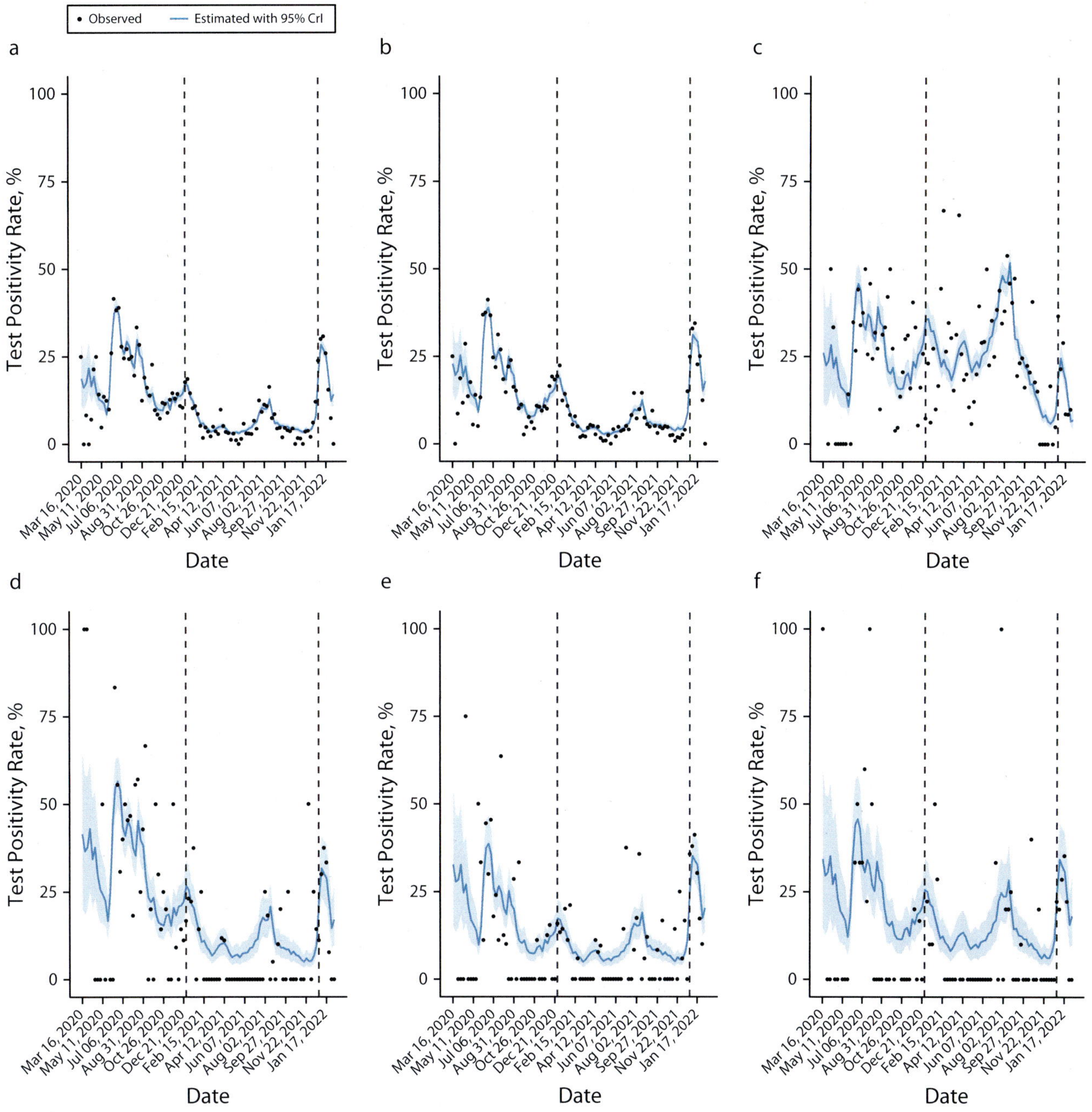

FIGURE 1— **Selected Areas With Observed COVID-19 Test Positivity Rate and Model-Based Estimates for (a) Area 1, (b) Area 2, (c) Area 3, (d) Area 4, (e) Area 5, and (f) Area 6: Cameron County, TX, March 2020–February 2022**

Note. CBG = census block group; CrI = credible interval; TPR = test positivity rate. TPR is shown by the black dots; 95% credible intervals is shown in the light blue shade. The vertical dashed line represents January 1 of years 2021 and 2022. Areas 1–2 represent CBGs with a relatively larger number of tests, and the fitted lines followed closely with the observed TPRs, with narrow 95% CrIs. For areas with sparse tests (areas 4–6), model-based estimates provided the needed shrinkage, which we obtained by borrowing information across space and time, where the extreme values in observed TPRs were shrunken to the overall average and resembled the general trend at the county level.

whether there are testing gaps. We provided valuable quantification of the additional tests needed. Fourth, our proposed spatial–temporal framework has the flexibility to accommodate the ever-changing dynamics related to COVID-19 when assessing testing disparity, which is particularly important.

The World Health Organization suggests that 10 to 30 tests should be performed for every positive case to control the spread of disease.[24,25] Such simple

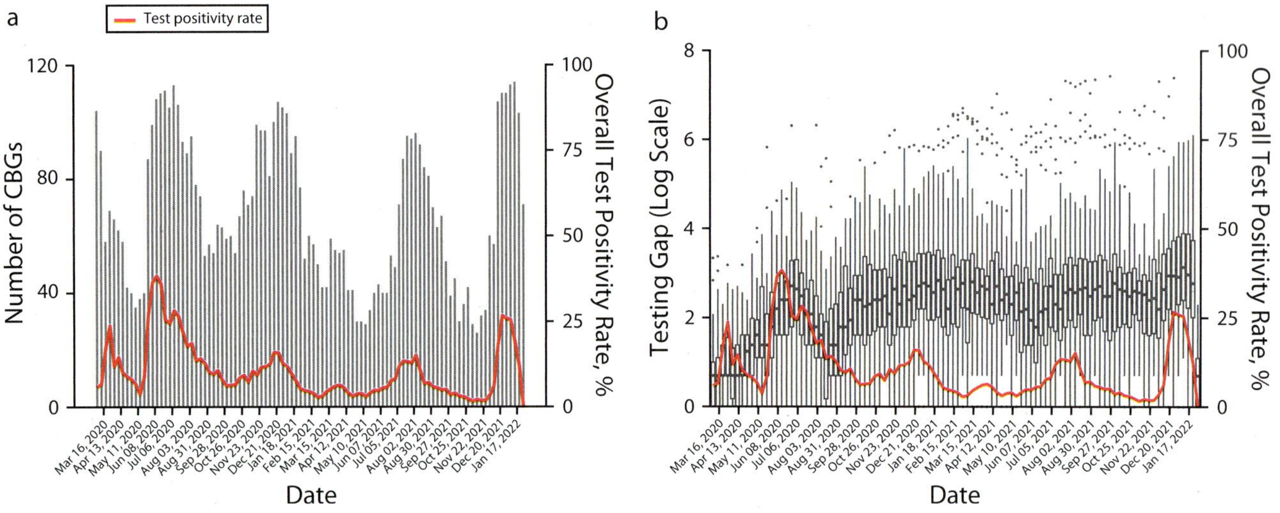

FIGURE 2— **Weekly Number of Tests Deficiency by (a) Number of CBGs, and (b) Testing Gap: Cameron County, TX, March 2020–February 2022**

Note. CBG = census block group. County-level overall test positivity rate was overlaid as the red line with the y-axis scale on the right. Panel a presents the number of CBGs that were identified with testing deficiency, by each week. Panel b presents the boxplots of the number of needed tests from these CBGs with testing deficiency. For example, 111 CBGs (of the total 222) experienced testing deficiency during the week of July 7, 2020 (panel a); among these CBGs, the additional needed tests had a median value of 410 and ranged from 1 and 548 (panel b).

calculations using the test and case ratio do not account for the changing intensity of the pandemic and may increase testing disparity across demographic subgroups or geographical areas. For example, CBGs that have not received sufficient tests would show lower infection rates, which would suggest even lower testing needs. More importantly, the ability of communities to implement the suggested number of tests depends on the availability of the tests, different tool kits, testing facility capacities, staffing, and many other factors. Finally, by using a Bayesian analytical framework, we were able to predict testing deficiency based on the local testing and infection patterns. This fills an important gap in the current research of SARS-CoV-2 testing disparities, in which testing gaps have always been identified retrospectively.

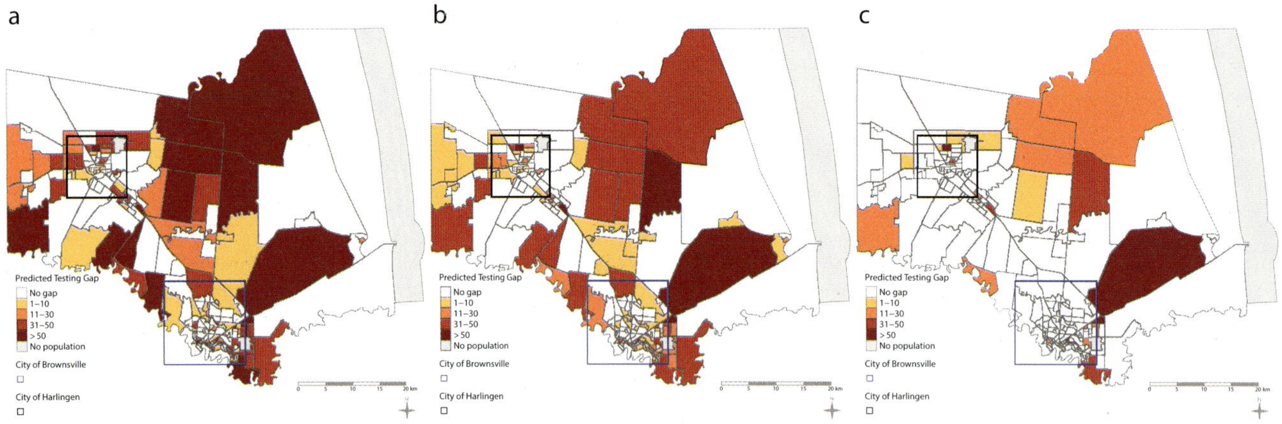

FIGURE 3— **Predicted Testing Disparity by Census Block Group for (a) Immediate Testing Deficiency, (b) Short-Term Testing Deficiency, and (c) Long-Term Testing Deficiency: Cameron County, TX, February 7–13, 2022**

Note. We used the observations before February 7, 2022, for comparison. Panel a presents the immediate testing deficiency, where testing rate was from the previous week (i.e., January 31–February 6, 2022) when performing the testing ranks. Panels b and c present the short-term testing deficiency using testing data from the previous month (i.e., January 10–February 6, 2022) and long-term testing deficiency using the average testing rate across the entire study period, respectively.

We argue that, in practice, the quantification of testing gap and deficiencies prospectively provides more useful and needed information for COVID-19 response.

Limitations

Our article has some limitations. First, we used only PCR-reported positive tests in our analysis. PCR is the most accurate SARS-CoV-2 testing method and, indeed, was used for the majority of the tests in the SARS-CoV-2 surveillance data used in this analysis. As other over-the-counter tests and testing methods become more available, testing results may not be captured in official epidemiologic surveillance databases, which will affect testing gap assessment. We consider this deficit a reporting issue commonly seen in surveillance systems. Purportedly, if every SARS-CoV-2 test result was captured by a surveillance database, our approach would be able to estimate the testing gap. Second, we were not able to incorporate the SARS-CoV-2 transmission modes and contact-tracing information in quantifying the needed tests, which would be highly informative in identifying who should be tested and where testing might be most convenient. However, as this pandemic has shown, contact-tracing data are extremely challenging to collect[26] and generally have been unavailable for analytical purposes at the population level. Third, about 10% of the testing records could not be geocoded, as they either had missing addresses or used a post office box.

Conclusions

From an implementation science perspective, we believe that our proposed analytical framework offers policymakers and practitioners a tool for understanding SARS-CoV-2 testing disparities in geographically small communities. Local public health officials and practitioners often desire spatial granularity, such as which street blocks they should go to for the community educational program or door-to-door visits to promote COVID-19 testing. Our proposed analytical framework provides a data-driven approach for this decision-making process. Community leaders, with this understanding and the knowledge of which small geographically bounded areas to prioritize, can address testing disparities with coordinated multilevel interventions by enhancing access to testing, improving outreach to assist in education and navigation to testing, and implementing effective large and small media messages to promote testing tailored to the population. Future research on the use of this approach and the derived data to drive these decisions should be rigorously evaluated to determine whether testing gaps across locations are eliminated in health disparate populations. AJPH

ABOUT THE AUTHORS

Cici Bauer, Xiaona Li, and Kehe Zhang are with the Department of Biostatistics and Data Science, School of Public Health, The University of Texas Health Science Center at Houston. Miryoung Lee, Susan Fisher-Hoch, and Joseph McCormick are with the Department of Epidemiology, Human Genetics and Environmental Science, School of Public Health, The University of Texas Health Science Center at Houston. Esmeralda Guajardo is with the Cameron County Public Health, San Benito, TX. Maria E. Fernandez and Belinda Reininger are with the Department of Health Promotion and Behavior Sciences, School of Public Health, The University of Texas Health Science Center at Houston.

CORRESPONDENCE

Correspondence should be sent to Cici Bauer, 1200 Pressler St, Houston, TX 77030 (e-mail: cici.x.bauer@uth.tmc.edu). Reprints can be ordered at http://www.ajph.org by clicking the "Reprints" link.

PUBLICATION INFORMATION

Full Citation: Bauer C, Li X, Zhang K, et al. A novel Bayesian spatial–temporal approach to quantify SARS-CoV-2 testing disparities for small area estimation. *Am J Public Health*. 2023;113(1):40–48.

Acceptance Date: September 10, 2022.

DOI: https://doi.org/10.2105/AJPH.2022.307127

CONTRIBUTORS

C. Bauer conceptualized and designed the analysis. C. Bauer, X. Li, and K. Zhang analyzed the data and wrote the initial draft of the article. M. Lee, E. Guajardo, and B. Reininger acquired the data. M. Lee, S. Fisher-Hoch, J. McCormick, M. E. Fernandez, and B. Reininger revised the article. M. E. Fernandez and B. Reininger acquired financial support for the project. All authors interpreted the results.

ACKNOWLEDGMENTS

This work was partially supported by the National Institutes of Health RADx–Underserved Populations (RADx–UP) initiative (grants 3UL1TR003167-02S1 and UL1 TR003167-02S6).

We acknowledge the important contribution of epidemiologists and staff in providing expertise, valuable feedback, and guidance during the revision from Cameron County Public Health. These staff include Daniel Piñon (health disparities epidemiologist), Raquel Castillo (chief epidemiologist), and Ashley Rui (health emergency preparedness program director). We also thank all the officials of the counties for their tireless efforts in setting up and operating testing facilities, software for COVID-19 testing appointments, and all the other work necessary in epidemic control.

CONFLICTS OF INTEREST

The authors report no conflicts of interest.

HUMAN PARTICIPANT PROTECTION

The University of Texas Health Science Center School of Public Health institutional review board approved this study (no. HSC-SPH-20-1372).

REFERENCES

1. Lieberman-Cribbin W, Alpert N, Flores R, Taioli E. Analyzing disparities in COVID-19 testing trends according to risk for COVID-19 severity across New York City. *BMC Public Health*. 2021;21(1):1717. https://doi.org/10.1186/s12889-021-11762-0
2. Adepoju OE, Ojinnaka CO. County-level determinants of COVID-19 testing and cases: are there racial/ethnic disparities in Texas? *Popul Health Manag*. 2021;24(5):589–594. https://doi.org/10.1089/pop.2020.0300
3. Kim HN, Lan KF, Nkyekyer E, et al. Assessment of disparities in COVID-19 testing and infection across language groups in Seattle, Washington. *JAMA Netw Open*. 2020;3(9):e2021213. https://doi.org/10.1001/jamanetworkopen.2020.21213
4. Reitsma MB, Claypool AL, Vargo J, et al. Racial/ethnic disparities in COVID-19 exposure risk, testing, and cases at the subcounty level in California. *Health Aff (Millwood)*. 2021;40(6):870–878. https://doi.org/10.1377/hlthaff.2021.00098
5. Ferguson JM, Justice AC, Osborne TF, Magid HSA, Purnell AL, Rentsch CT. Geographic and temporal

variation in racial and ethnic disparities in SARS-CoV-2 positivity between February 2020 and August 2021 in the United States. *Sci Rep.* 2022;12(1):273. https://doi.org/10.1038/s41598-021-03967-5

6. Farmer B. Racial disparities emerge in Tennessee's testing for COVID-19. April 1, 2020. Available at: https://wpln.org/post/racial-disparities-emerge-in-tennessees-testing-for-covid-19. Accessed April 22, 2022.
7. Tan TQ, Kullar R, Swartz TH, Mathew TA, Piggott DA, Berthaud V. Location matters: geographic disparities and impact of coronavirus disease 2019. *J Infect Dis.* 2020;222(12):1951–1954. https://doi.org/10.1093/infdis/jiaa583
8. Dryden-Peterson S, Velásquez GE, Stopka TJ, Davey S, Lockman S, Ojikutu BO. Disparities in SARS-CoV-2 Testing in Massachusetts During the COVID-19 Pandemic. *JAMA Netw Open.* 2021;4(2):e2037067. [Erratum in: *JAMA Netw Open.* 2021;4(4):e2110970]. https://doi.org/10.1001/jamanetworkopen.2020.37067
9. Rao JNK. *Isabel Molina. Small Area Estimation.* Hoboken, NJ: John Wiley; 2015. Available at: https://onlinelibrary.wiley.com/doi/book/10.1002/9781118735855. Accessed March 26, 2022
10. US Census Bureau QuickFacts. 2020. Available at: https://www.census.gov/quickfacts. Accessed November 11, 2022.
11. RADx-UP. About RADx-UP. Available at: https://radx-up.org/about. Accessed April 22, 2022.
12. Knorr-Held L. Bayesian modelling of inseparable space–time variation in disease risk. *Stat Med.* 2000;19(17–18):2555–2567.
13. Bauer C, Wakefield J, Rue H, Self S, Feng Z, Wang Y. Bayesian penalized spline models for the analysis of spatio-temporal count data. *Stat Med.* 2016;35(11):1848–1865. https://doi.org/10.1002/sim.6785
14. Saavedra P, Santana A, Bello L, Pacheco JM, Sanjuán E. A Bayesian spatio-temporal analysis of mortality rates in Spain: application to the COVID-19 2020 outbreak. *Popul Health Metr.* 2021;19(1):27. https://doi.org/10.1186/s12963-021-00259-y
15. Chen C, Wakefield J, Lumely T. The use of sampling weights in Bayesian hierarchical models for small area estimation. *Spat Spatiotemporal Epidemiol.* 2014;11:33–43. https://doi.org/10.1016/j.sste.2014.07.002
16. Mercer L, Wakefield J, Chen C, Lumley T. A comparison of spatial smoothing methods for small area estimation with sampling weights. *Spat Stat.* 2014;8:69–85. https://doi.org/10.1016/j.spasta.2013.12.001
17. Besag J, York J, Mollié A. Bayesian image restoration, with two applications in spatial statistics. *Ann Inst Stat Math.* 1991;43(1):1–20. https://doi.org/10.1007/BF00116466
18. Gelfand AE, Dey DK. Bayesian model choice: asymptotics and exact calculations. *J R Stat Soc B.* 1994;56(3):501–514. https://doi.org/10.1111/j.2517-6161.1994.tb01996.x
19. Lieberman-Cribbin W, Tuminello S, Flores RM, Taioli E. Disparities in COVID-19 testing and positivity in New York City. *Am J Prev Med.* 2020;59(3):326–332. https://doi.org/10.1016/j.amepre.2020.06.005
20. Rue H, Martino S, Chopin N. Approximate Bayesian inference for latent Gaussian models by using integrated nested Laplace approximations. *J R Stat Soc Series B Stat Methodol.* 2009;71(2):319–392. https://doi.org/10.1111/j.1467-9868.2008.00700.x
21. Fisher-Hoch SP, Rentfro AR, Salinas JJ, et al. Socioeconomic status and prevalence of obesity and diabetes in a Mexican American community, Cameron County, Texas, 2004–2007. *Prev Chronic Dis.* 2010;7(3):A53.
22. Fisher-Hoch SP, Vatcheva KP, Rahbar MH, McCormick JB. Undiagnosed diabetes and pre-diabetes in health disparities. *PLoS One.* 2015;10(7):e0133135. https://doi.org/10.1371/journal.pone.0133135
23. Watt GP, Fisher-Hoch SP, Rahbar MH, et al. Mexican American and South Asian population-based cohorts reveal high prevalence of type 2 diabetes and crucial differences in metabolic phenotypes. *BMJ Open Diabetes Res Care.* 2018;6(1):e000436. https://doi.org/10.1136/bmjdrc-2017-000436
24. Mody A, Pfeifauf K, Bradley C, et al. Understanding drivers of coronavirus disease 2019 (COVID-19) racial disparities: a population-level analysis of COVID-19 testing among Black and White populations. *Clin Infect Dis.* 2021;73(9):e2921–e2931. https://doi.org/10.1093/cid/ciaa1848
25. Siddarth D, Katz R, Graeden E, Allen D, Lumely T. Evidence roundup: why positive test rates need to fall below 3%. May 29, 2020. Available at: https://globalhealth.harvard.edu/evidence-roundup-why-positive-test-rates-need-to-fall-below-3. Accessed March 10, 2022.
26. Megnin-Viggars O, Carter P, Melendez-Torres GJ, Weston D, Rubin GJ. Facilitators and barriers to engagement with contact tracing during infectious disease outbreaks: a rapid review of the evidence. *PLoS One.* 2020;15(10):e0241473. https://doi.org/10.1371/journal.pone.0241473

The Sequential Multiple Assignment Randomized Trial for Controlling Infectious Diseases: A Review of Recent Developments

Xinru Wang, MS, and Bibhas Chakraborty, PhD

See also Vaughan, p. 35, Seewald, p. 37, Bauer et al., p. 40, and Liu et al., p. 60.

Infectious diseases have posed severe threats to public health across the world. Effective prevention and control of infectious diseases in the long term requires adapting interventions based on epidemiological evidence. The sequential multiple assignment randomized trial (SMART) is a multistage randomized trial that can provide valid evidence of when and how to adapt interventions for controlling infectious diseases based on evolving epidemiological evidence.

We review recent developments in SMARTs to bring wider attention to the potential benefits of employing SMARTs in constructing effective adaptive interventions for controlling infectious diseases and other threats to public health. We discuss 2 example SMARTs for infectious diseases and summarize recent developments in SMARTs from the varied aspects of design, analysis, cost, and ethics.

Public health investigators are encouraged to familiarize themselves with the related materials we discuss and collaborate with experts in SMARTs to translate the methodological developments into preeminent public health research. (*Am J Public Health*. 2023;113(1):49–59. https://doi.org/10.2105/AJPH.2022.307135)

AJPH January 2023, Vol 113, No. 1

Infectious diseases have posed severe threats to public health throughout human history. In recent years, the COVID-19 pandemic has inflicted enormous human suffering and in tandem has attracted considerable research attention. To slow the spread of COVID-19 and to reduce the morbidity and mortality rates, numerous interventions have been imposed to control the spread of the disease (e.g., limiting group size of social gatherings, promoting vaccine uptake, and issuing stay-at-home orders).[1] However, to minimize the negative impact on people's livelihood while also effectively controlling the diseases, decision-makers are required to find the precise ways to adapt health promotion and disease prevention programs based on evolving epidemiological evidence, instead of sticking to "one-size-fits-all" interventions.

Such sequences of decision-making about when and how to adapt interventions based on evolving epidemiological evidence have been widely applied to the prevention of infectious diseases and can be referred to as "adaptive interventions," also known as "dynamic treatment regimens" or "adaptive treatment strategies" in the field of biostatistics.[2] The main components of an adaptive intervention are (1) intervention options, such as different types of interventions, delivery approaches, and dosage levels; (2) decision points, that is, the prespecified time points to recommend interventions based on baseline characteristics or intermediate tailoring variables; (3) tailoring variables, that is, variables that can be used to identify which intervention should be recommended and for whom (e.g., mediators, moderators, or early surrogates for longer-term outcomes of interest); and (4) decision rules, that is, prespecified rules that can recommend interventions based on previous historical data.

One example of an adaptive intervention for treating COVID-19–positive patients with mild symptoms is the following: First, treat the patients at community care facilities with general medical care. Then, assign patients who respond adequately, according to prespecified criteria, to the community recovery facilities before discharging them, and hospitalize nonresponders and provide intensified medical care.[3]

With the increasing popularity of adaptive interventions, there appears to be a wave of interest in developing a promising evidence-based adaptive intervention to maximize patient gains.[4] When faced with life-threatening infectious diseases, researchers rely primarily on historical experiences and observational data to inform decision-making procedures, given that explanatory randomized controlled trials (RCTs) are time consuming and may fail to generate up-to-date conclusions to guide the implementation of public health interventions. However, the validity of such an analysis based on observational data depends on the untestable ignorable intervention assignment assumption, that is, the assumption that receiving the intervention or not is independent of the potential outcomes.[5]

At the outset of the COVID-19 pandemic, observational studies were essential to provide evidence for prompt public policies. However, as the increasing level of COVID-19 vaccine coverage has significantly decreased the morbidity and mortality rates, proactive research (e.g., pragmatic study designs) is needed to move to the next-generation epidemiological prevention measures and further identify evidence-based interventions for future public health practice for infectious diseases.

The sequential multiple assignment randomized trial (SMART) is an experimental design consisting of multiple randomization stages.[2] This type of design serves as a promising tool to address scientific questions about constructing effective adaptive interventions for controlling infectious diseases. SMARTs have been implemented in various health domains, including diet and weight control,[6] HIV infection,[7] mental health,[8] and behavioral sciences.[9] This recent surge in the prevalence of SMARTs can be attributed to the increasingly ripened methodology in the design and analysis aspects and the availability of some good tutorial articles providing blow-by-blow guidance to help practitioners gain a better understanding of SMARTs.[10–16] However, to the best of our knowledge, except for the setting of HIV infection, there are far fewer SMARTs in the field of infectious diseases, likely on the grounds that contagious diseases require a rapid real-time response at the early stage of the outbreak. Furthermore, SMARTs may be relatively uncommon to many public health researchers; thus, researchers may hesitate to choose a SMART design when constructing evidence-based adaptive interventions for controlling infectious diseases.

We aim to facilitate the implementation of SMARTs for infectious diseases by summarizing the recent developments in SMARTs with a special focus on infectious diseases. We first review 2 SMARTs for infectious diseases to help readers gain a better grasp of employing SMARTs to improve public health. We then provide details about associated data analysis and cost and ethical considerations in SMARTs. We also summarize the existing software for designing and analyzing SMARTs to build a bridge between methodological developments and practical implementation. Although we focus on infectious diseases, our discussion is sufficiently general to apply SMARTs to a wide range of other fields.

EXAMPLE SMARTS FOR INFECTIOUS DISEASES

In this section, we provide 2 example SMARTs for controlling infectious diseases.

Example 1

Despite the high global capacity to produce COVID-19 vaccines and the increasing clinical trial data demonstrating their effectiveness, some people still hesitate to get vaccinated because they fear potentially severe side effects or simply lack the conviction that the vaccines are useful. Governments have taken public measures (e.g., mounting public media programs) to dispel the rumors about COVID-19 vaccines. However, such measures can reach only a limited audience. More efforts are needed to further promote vaccine uptake and speed up the process of herd immunity.

There is a large-scale SMART, each stage of which was planned as a separate RCT for investigating the effect of digital interventions on the uptake of COVID-19 vaccines.[17] The investigators in this SMART considered several first-line interventions to motivate people to get vaccinated and second-line interventions to further remind those who have not received the first vaccine dose in a prespecified period because of having received the first-line intervention. A simplified version of the design is presented in Figure 1. Participants who had not already taken the first dose at the starting point of the trial

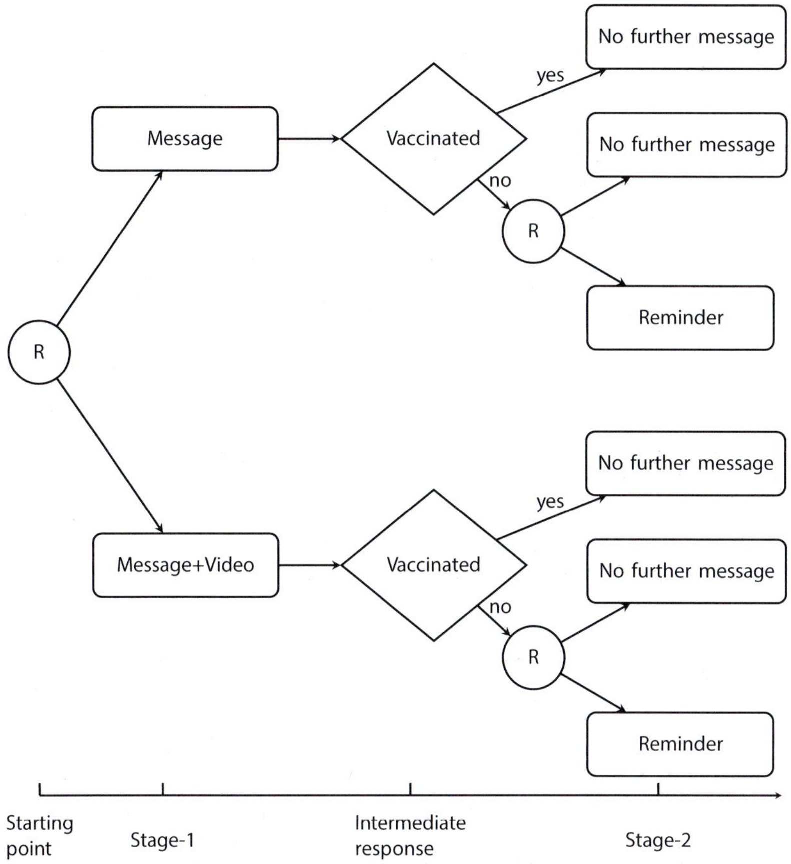

FIGURE 1— A SMART for Developing Digital Adaptive Interventions to Facilitate the Uptake of COVID-19 Vaccines

Note. R = randomization.

were equally randomized to either the message group or the message plus video group. After 8 days, those who still had not received the first dose were randomized to either the no further message group or the reminder group, with a reminder message that could help clear potential barriers to vaccination, such as forgetfulness, hassle, costs, and procrastination. The primary outcome of interest was whether a participant has made the appointment for the first vaccine dose. There were 4 adaptive interventions embedded in this SMART: (1) first send a motivating message, then send a basic reminder message if not vaccinated; (2) send a motivating message only at the starting point; (3) first send a motivating message plus explanatory video, then send a reminder message if not vaccinated; and (4) send a motivating message plus explanatory video only at the starting point.

Example 2

Malaria, a potentially serious infectious disease transmitted by a specific type of mosquito, can be effectively controlled by the use of long-lasting insecticide-treated nets (LLIN), indoor residual spraying (IRS), and larval source management (LSM).[18] The high cost of implementing IRS and LSM is a major concern that needs to be considered when constructing an effective adaptive intervention for malaria control, and more scientific evidence is required to guide the prevention interventions, such as when and how to employ IRS and LSM while ensuring efficient harnessing of the resources for malaria control.

An ongoing cluster-randomized SMART (Figure 2) was designed to collect evidence for constructing an effective adaptive intervention for malaria control in western Kenya.[18] By "cluster randomized," we mean that the interventions are randomly administered at the cluster level (e.g., a village or several neighboring villages), whereas the outcomes are collected at the individual level (i.e., residents in the randomly selected households). The enrolled clusters are randomized to receive LLIN, piperonyl butoxide (PBO) LLIN (the next-generation LLIN combining the synergist piperonyl butoxide with pyrethroids), or the combination of LLIN and IRS. After 15 months, clusters will be evaluated for the response status based on the change in clinical malaria incidence when using PBO LLIN or LLIN + IRS compared with LLIN alone. Responders will continue with their initial intervention, whereas nonresponders to PBO LLIN are randomized to the combination of PBO LLIN + LSM or the intervention determined by a reinforcement learning algorithm developed to generate unbalanced randomization probabilities in favor of the estimated superior intervention for each cluster, and nonresponders to LLIN + IRS are randomized to LLIN + IRS + LSM or PBO LLIN + IRS. The primary outcome of interest is the clinical malaria incidence. The primary aim of this trial is to compare first-line interventions PBO LLIN and LLIN + IRS in terms of the effectiveness of reducing malaria incidence after 36 months, and the secondary aim is to identify the

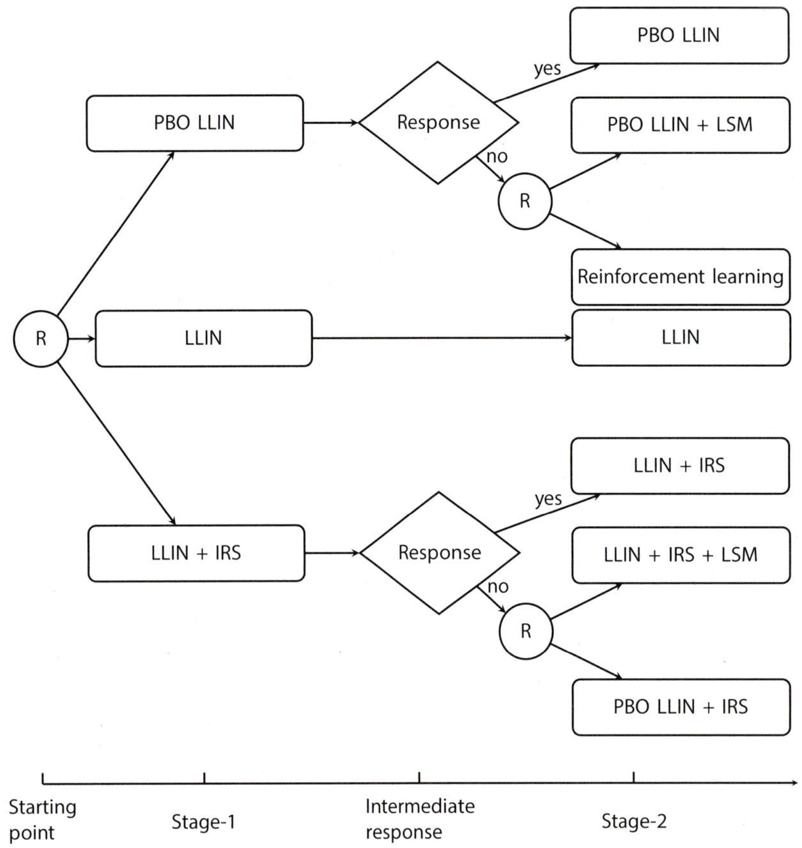

FIGURE 2— A SMART for Developing Optimal Adaptive Interventions for Malaria Control

Note. IRS = indoor residual spraying; LLIN = long-lasting insecticide-treated nets; LSM = larval source management; PBO = piperonyl butoxide; R = randomization.

most effective intervention to reduce malaria incidence.

In addition to these 2 examples, there is another ongoing SMART for developing an optimal adaptive intervention to facilitate COVID-19 testing and adherence to the Centers for Disease Control and Prevention recommendations among high-risk people in an urban community.[19] We have not presented details here because of space limitations.

WHEN TO USE SMARTS

There have been tremendous improvements in the experimental designs for constructing interventions with multiple components, such as factorial designs,[20] SMARTs, and microrandomized trials.[21] Given that the concepts of these designs are somewhat entangled, researchers may be confused about when to use SMARTs at the beginning of the design stage, which limits the broader use of SMARTs. With this backdrop, Nahum-Shani et al.[22] proposed a practical framework to provide valuable insights into choosing the most appropriate design among all these candidate designs. To briefly summarize, a SMART design is a proper choice when (1) the interventions of interest are multicomponent interventions, (2) the researchers aim to select multiple effective components out of all candidates to be included in the final intervention, (3) there are research interests in the timing of intervention components, and (4) the conditions are changing slowly.

It is important to note that, in cases in which all 4 conditions for choosing SMARTs are met, multiple single-stage RCTs may serve as an alternative way to examine the effect of the initial and subsequent interventions.[23] Single-stage RCTs, however, have some inevitable disadvantages compared with SMARTs.[11] First, single-stage RCTs do not allow researchers to investigate either the synergetic effect between the initial and subsequent interventions in the long term or the potential tailoring variables for more tailored adaptive interventions.

In addition, it can be argued that participants in SMARTs may be less likely to drop out because alternative interventions are provided in cases of insufficient early response. In other words, SMARTs provide participants with a "safety net" (i.e., a second chance to get a different, potentially beneficial intervention when the current intervention is not working). By contrast, with single-stage RCTs, participants with apparently ineffective interventions have no choice but to discontinue the intervention or drop out. SMARTs can also be replaced by an up-front randomized trial,[24] which randomizes patients to candidate adaptive interventions at the beginning of the study. Compared with SMARTs, the rationale and statistical methods in up-front randomized trials are easier to understand. However, several studies have demonstrated that the estimators from SMARTs are more efficient (with smaller variance) than are those from up-front randomized trials.[24,25] Moreover, rerandomizations in SMARTs allow restratification, which may be useful in achieving balanced distributions of covariates in rerandomizations, whereas up-front randomized trials do not allow this.

SAMPLE SIZE CALCULATIONS IN SMARTS

The required sample size in a SMART is dictated by its primary research questions.

Table 1 summarizes the most common primary goals of SMARTs, and some illustrative applications and software are provided for each case when applicable. Briefly, there are mainly 4 primary research goals in SMARTs: (1) performing the pilot evaluation, (2) estimating the main effects of first-line and second-line interventions, (3) comparing embedded adaptive interventions, and (4) developing the optimization goal (i.e., more deeply tailored adaptive interventions).

The evaluation of feasibility is often the intended goal in a pilot SMART, in which researchers assess the acceptability and the rationale of the embedded adaptive interventions as well as the fidelity of the study staff to implement the specified adaptive interventions in preparation for a future full-scale SMART. Almirall et al.[12] described in detail how to design a pilot SMART and proposed a feasibility-based method to determine the required sample size that ensures sufficient participants in each intervention sequence, allowing researchers to gather comprehensive information about the feasibility of a planned SMART. Building on this, Yan et al.[26] presented a precision-based method to size a pilot SMART with various types of outcomes, by which the SEs of estimates of interest are confined in a prespecified range.

TABLE 1— **Sample Size Calculations for Different Primary Research Questions in SMARTs**

Primary Goal	Method	Cluster/Individual	Primary Outcome	Example Trials	Software
Pilot evaluation	Precision based	Individual	Continuous/binary/count[26]	Yan et al.[27]	https://bit.ly/3zyktU7
	Feasibility based	Both	All[12]	Lambert et al.[28]	https://bit.ly/3Nqq3gY
Main effect	Effect of first-line treatments	Similar to RCTs	Similar to RCTs[29]	Zhou et al.[18]	https://bit.ly/3SUgcRG
	Effect of second-line treatments	Similar to RCTs	Similar to RCTs[29]	Sherwood et al.[6]	https://bit.ly/3SUgcRG
Compare adaptive interventions	Select optimal adaptive interventions	Individual	Continuous[29]		
	Pairwise superiority testing	Individual	Continuous[29–31]		https://bit.ly/3SUgcRG https://bit.ly/3Fx1blQ[32]
			Continuous/binary[33]		
			Binary[34]		https://bit.ly/3SUgcRG
			Survival[35]		
			Continuous longitudinal[36]		
			Ordinal[37]		https://bit.ly/3NmHeQA
		Cluster	Continuous/binary[33]	Quanbeck et al.[38]	
			Continuous[39]		
			Continuous (skew-t, MNAR)[40]		https://bit.ly/3zwLTtA[41]
	Pairwise noninferiority testing	Individual	Continuous[42]		https://bit.ly/3Wnd7gf
	MCB testing	Individual	Continuous[43]		https://bit.ly/3DK1EyT[44]
			Binary[45]		https://bit.ly/3Nluw4R, https://bit.ly/3NvA1Os[46]
Optimization	Normality based or projection based	Individual	Continuous[47]		

Note. MCB = multiple comparisons with the best; MNAR = missing not at random; RCT = randomized controlled trial; SMART = sequential multiple assignment randomized trial.

For a full-fledged SMART, one of the most common primary research goals that drive sample size calculation is to investigate the effect of individual components. Oetting et al.[29] gave a detailed illustration of deriving the required sample size for comparing stage-specific intervention effects with continuous primary outcomes. Briefly, the calculation procedure is similar to that used in RCTs, except that the response rate of initial interventions should be incorporated when investigating the intervention effect of subsequent interventions for responders and nonresponders. Practitioners can follow the same principles for other types of primary outcomes.

A sizable literature focuses on comparing embedded adaptive interventions as a whole, comparing 2 or more embedded adaptive interventions,[29–31] or screening out the inferior set of adaptive interventions.[43] Ghosh et al.[42] further extended the framework by emphasizing the importance of noninferiority testing between 2 embedded adaptive interventions to construct an almost equally effective adaptive intervention with lower cost, less burden, or fewer side effects and developed the analysis and sample size calculation formulas for the noninferiority testing. All the aforementioned sample size calculation methods are suitable for individual-level SMARTs with continuous primary outcomes. Recently there has been tremendous progress in deriving the sample size calculation formulas for comparing embedded adaptive interventions in individual-level SMARTs with binary,[34] survival,[35,48–50] ordinal,[37] and continuous longitudinal[36] outcomes; for cluster-level SMARTs with binary and continuous outcomes[33,39]; and for cluster-level SMARTs with various features of outcomes, including spatial clustering, non-Gaussianity, and missing not at random.[40]

Investigators may also be interested in constructing more tailored adaptive interventions (i.e., sequences of decision rules that recommend intervention options based on additional observed information; e.g., baseline characteristics or intermediate potential tailoring variables). The research question is thus to explore an optimal tailored adaptive intervention that is expected to maximize the overall effectiveness of interventions if applied to the entire study population. Although optimization is a possible primary goal, it often serves as a bonus on top of investigating main effects and comparing embedded adaptive interventions when conducting a SMART.

When a SMART is designed with the optimization objective, the sample size calculation involves technical issues posed by estimating and evaluating an optimal adaptive intervention using the same data. Rose et al.[47] proposed normality-based and projection-based sample size calculation methods to ensure enough power for comparing the estimated optimal deeply tailored adaptive intervention with the fixed standard intervention. Note that the required sample size for comparing embedded adaptive interventions or optimization is often higher than that for comparing stage-specific interventions. Researchers are advised to define the primary goals of SMARTs based on the research budget for recruiting participants and the major research questions of interest.

Although significant strides have been made in statistical methodology, to the best of our knowledge, these sample size calculation methods for comparing adaptive interventions or optimizations are scarcely used in real practice. The reason for this may be that both the scientific investigators and the statisticians are more familiar with the statistical methods in standard trials, so they are inclined to sizing SMARTs based on the main effect, with the additional goal of comparing embedded adaptive interventions or optimization to provide complementary information for future confirmatory trials. More efforts are needed to translate the developed methodologies to real clinical and public health practice by lucidly explaining the concepts of SMARTs and the statistical tools to a broader audience.

DATA ANALYSIS IN SMARTS

When the research question concerns examining the main effects in a SMART, standard statistical methods in RCTs can be used to analyze the SMART data. However, when the goal is to discern the effectiveness of 2 or more embedded adaptive interventions, adjustments to the standard methods are required to account for the sequential randomizations in SMARTs. The weighted and replicated regression[51] can provide valid inferences of the mean outcomes of all the embedded adaptive interventions simultaneously, by weighting and replicating observations to account for the underrepresentation of certain subgroups because of the design of the trial. Nahum-Shani et al.[52] presented a thorough guideline on how to use this method to analyze data from SMARTs with end-of-study continuous outcomes. This method holds the promise of being straightforward and accessible to practitioners as it is akin to standard regression

TABLE 2— R Packages for Data Analysis in SMART

Package Name	Objective	Outcome	Method	Software
SMARTAR[32]	Comparisons between embedded adaptive interventions	Continuous, binary	Global/pairwise testing	https://bit.ly/3Fx1blQ
DTR[60]	Comparisons between embedded adaptive interventions	Survival	Weighted logrank tests	https://bit.ly/3NvMyBl
DTRlearn2[61]	Optimization	Continuous, binary	Q-learning, other outcome-weighted learning methods	https://bit.ly/3zxCwK5
DTRreg[62]	Optimization	Continuous, binary, survival	Q-learning, G-estimation, dynamic weighted ordinary least squares (dWOLS)	https://bit.ly/3zypg83
DynTxRegime[63]	Optimization	Continuous, binary	Q-learning, interactive Q-learning, weighted learning, value-search methods	https://bit.ly/3WlZGx2

Note. SMART = sequential multiple assignment randomized trial.

methods and can be executed using standard software. The method has been extended to analyze data from SMARTs with continuous longitudinal outcomes,[53] binary outcomes,[34] and continuous outcomes in cluster-level SMARTs,[39] and it has been employed in real practice for primary, secondary, and exploratory analyses.[6,54,55]

Q-learning, a stage-by-stage regression-type procedure,[56] can be used to identify an optimal deeply tailored adaptive intervention (as opposed to the embedded adaptive interventions) based on SMART data. The letter Q stands for the quality of an intervention (e.g., a desired clinical outcome), conditional on the observed information and subsequent interventions. Intuitively, Q-learning begins by estimating the optimal decision rule at the last stage and moves backward successively to construct an optimal decision rule at each stage, assuming the use of optimal decision rules at the subsequent stages. Nahum-Shani et al.[56] provide a detailed illustration of implementing Q-learning to construct more tailored adaptive interventions in SMARTs. Other notable statistical learning–based and tree-based methods[57–59] can also be applied to develop optimal adaptive interventions. Table 2 lists several user-friendly R packages to compare embedded adaptive interventions or develop more tailored adaptive interventions.

Missing data problems pose a significant challenge to data analysis in SMARTs. Standard imputation methods cannot be directly applied to deal with missing data in SMARTs because of the nonstandard multistage randomization procedure. However, researchers can alleviate the impact of missing data on the validity of analysis from both design and analysis perspectives. First, as stated by Almirall et al.,[12] pilot SMARTs can provide valuable insights for future full-scale SMARTs in terms of strategies to reduce the dropout rate and to treat early dropout patients. Liu et al.[64] presented a SMART with enrichment to improve design efficiency when the dropout rate is high by augmenting the trial sample with new patients who have received previous stages' interventions. In terms of analysis, Shortreed et al.[65] proposed a multiple imputation strategy to tackle the unique missing data problems arising in SMARTs. Researchers are encouraged to employ these tactics to achieve more reliable inferences from SMARTs and perform sensitivity analysis to check the validity of the missing at random assumption.

COST-EFFECTIVE ADAPTIVE INTERVENTIONS

Effective control of infectious diseases requires the involvement of a variety of communities and stakeholders. Efficient use of scarce medical and financial resources is one of the major challenges when implementing large-scale prevention and intervention programs.[66] When intervention resources are limited for conducting a SMART, the optimal allocation of interventions with a fixed budget constraint is desired. Morciano and Moerbeek[67] proposed an optimal allocation strategy for simultaneously comparing embedded adaptive interventions in SMARTs with a fixed sample size or a fixed budget and provided an easy to use Web app to facilitate the use of this optimal allocation strategy.

Although the efficacy of improving outcomes is often the main focus when developing optimal adaptive interventions, the cost of an intervention is another important factor to consider in health economics. When an intervention is more effective and less costly than another, it is deemed to be the strictly superior intervention. However, if the more effective intervention costs more, to select the adaptive interventions that can be both effective and sustainable in practice, policymakers are expected to weigh their options between health efficacy and the additional cost per unit outcome improvement. Xu et al.[68] proposed a decision tree–based algorithm to develop a cost-effective adaptive intervention with the net monetary benefit as the primary outcome. This cost-effectiveness analysis method is recognized as a promising way to analyze SMART data and develop more tailored cost-effective adaptive interventions. As it has been widely acknowledged that cost effectiveness is a major concern during clinical practice, researchers are encouraged to collect cost-related data for a future cost-effectiveness analysis.

ETHICAL CONSIDERATIONS IN SMARTS

Even though SMARTs can potentially unpack the black box of sequenced multicomponent interventions, they may require more time to implement than do standard RCTs. For infectious diseases, however, the earlier the intervention is delivered, the more benefits it will provide for public health. With the aim of reducing the time for conducting SMARTs, Wu et al.[69] proposed a SMART with interim monitoring, in which the global hypothesis testing of all embedded adaptive interventions is conducted at each interim monitoring time, and early stopping of the trial is permitted if the evidence of efficacy is sufficient.

When faced with emerging infectious diseases that threaten millions of human lives, it is imperative to conduct trials to select effective interventions for future patients while minimizing the infection and mortality rate of enrolled participants. Several extensions of SMARTs can be potentially applied to increase the number of participants receiving the optimal intervention in SMARTs for controlling infectious diseases. Cheung et al.[70] provided a SMART with adaptive randomization based on Q-learning. Roughly speaking, it estimates the parameters of the stage-specific conditional mean outcomes based on the data from previous patients and updates the assignment probabilities in favor of the interventions with higher values of the predicted stage-specific conditional mean outcomes. Wang et al.[71] presented a response-adaptive SMART to incorporate the short-term intervention efficacy shown from previous patients when randomizing the stage 2 interventions. So far, very few adaptive SMARTs have been implemented in practice; for example, Ruppert et al.[72] presented a trial protocol for a SMART with an interim analysis targeting older patients with chronic lymphocytic leukemia, in which rerandomization will be discontinued if the adaptive intervention to be randomized has proven to be inferior to the others.

At the early stage of an infectious disease outbreak, the information regarding potentially effective interventions accumulates continuously, and as a result, a more flexible trial design that allows adding new interventions and removing inferior interventions may be a better choice to save on costs and time. One of the most notable examples is the RECOVERY (Randomized Evaluation of COVid-19 ThERapY) trial,[73] a platform trial to discover effective interventions to reduce the mortality rate in hospitalized COVID-19 patients. Future work could extend SMARTs to have such flexibility and compare its statistical properties with other types of SMARTs, which may be useful in planning for future pandemic control.

CONCLUSIONS

We sought to facilitate the application of SMARTs in the area of infectious diseases by familiarizing interested investigators with the general framework of SMARTs and the recent developments in SMARTs in terms of methodology and practical guidelines. Despite our best efforts to find related literature for a thorough review, there may be some publications that we have missed. Although we do not provide an exhaustive list of related articles, we cover the most important aspects of conducting a SMART, from identifying scenarios in which SMARTs are applicable and summarizing design and analysis methods for SMARTs to addressing the costs and ethical issues in such trials. Note that we did not intend to provide step-by-step guidance on implementing a SMART; instead, we attempted to provide comprehensive resources for potential designers of SMARTs for infectious diseases, including example SMART designs for controlling infectious diseases and easy to use software for sample size calculation and data analysis in SMARTs.

Although SMARTs may seem conceptually complex to some readers, they can shift the fixed interventions to the more realistic interventions in which modifying interventions is allowed according to the early response status, which mimics what public health practitioners do in practice. We hope that investigators will draw inspiration from this review and translate it into practice to improve public health in the face of life-threatening infectious diseases as well as other potential health-related challenges. AJPH

ABOUT THE AUTHORS

Xinru Wang and Bibhas Chakraborty are with the Centre for Quantitative Medicine, Duke-NUS Medical School, Singapore. Bibhas Chakraborty is also with the Department of Statistics and Data Science, National University of Singapore, Singapore.

CORRESPONDENCE

Correspondence should be sent to Bibhas Chakraborty, the Centre for Quantitative Medicine and the Program in Health Services and Systems Research, Duke-NUS Medical School, 8 College Rd, Level 6, #06-31, Singapore 169857 (e-mail: bibhas.chakraborty@duke-nus.edu.sg). Reprints can be ordered at http://www.ajph.org by clicking the "Reprints" link.

PUBLICATION INFORMATION

Full Citation: Wang X, Chakraborty B. The sequential multiple assignment randomized trial for controlling infectious diseases: a review of recent developments. *Am J Public Health*. 2023;113(1): 49–59.

Acceptance Date: September 19, 2022.

DOI: https://doi.org/10.2105/AJPH.2022.307135

CONTRIBUTORS

X. Wang drafted and revised the article.
B. Chakraborty helped write and critically revise the article.

ACKNOWLEDGMENTS

B. Chakraborty would like to acknowledge research support from a Khoo Bridge Funding Award (Duke-NUS-KBrFA/2021/0040) and a start-up grant from Duke-NUS Medical School, National University of Singapore.

We wish to acknowledge helpful comments from Roger Vaughan, DrPH, MS, and the anonymous reviewers.

CONFLICTS OF INTEREST

The authors have no conflicts of interest to declare.

HUMAN PARTICIPANT PROTECTION

No protocol approval was needed for this study because no human participants were involved.

REFERENCES

1. Brauner JM, Mindermann S, Sharma M, et al. Inferring the effectiveness of government interventions against COVID-19. *Science*. 2021;371(6531): eabd9338. https://doi.org/10.1126/science.abd9338
2. Murphy SA. An experimental design for the development of adaptive treatment strategies. *Stat Med*. 2005;24(10):1455–1481. https://doi.org/10.1002/sim.2022
3. Zhang J, Chua QHA, Shen XM, Viseikumaran JA, Teoh T, Tan NG. A Systematic implementation of telemedicine in Singapore's COVID-19 community recovery facilities. *Telemed E-Health*. 2022; Epub ahead of print. https://doi.org/10.1089/tmj.2021.0466
4. Lavori PW, Dawson R, Rush AJ. Flexible treatment strategies in chronic disease: clinical and research implications. *Biol Psychiatry*. 2000;48(6): 605–614. https://doi.org/10.1016/S0006-3223(00)00946-X
5. Rubin DB. Estimating causal effects of treatments in randomized and nonrandomized studies. *J Educ Psychol*. 1974;66(5):688–701. https://doi.org/10.1037/h0037350
6. Sherwood NE, Crain AL, Seburg EM, et al. BestFIT sequential multiple assignment randomized trial results: a SMART approach to developing individualized weight loss treatment sequences. *Ann Behav Med*. 2022;56(3):291–304. https://doi.org/10.1093/abm/kaab061
7. Mustanski B, Moskowitz DA, Moran KO, et al. Evaluation of a stepped-care eHealth HIV prevention program for diverse adolescent men who have sex with men: protocol for a hybrid type 1 effectiveness implementation trial of SMART. *JMIR Res Protoc*. 2020;9(8):e19701. https://doi.org/10.2196/19701
8. Schoenfelder EN, Chronis-Tuscano A, Strickland J, Almirall D, Stein MA. Piloting a sequential, multiple assignment, randomized trial for mothers with attention-deficit/hyperactivity disorder and their at-risk young children. *J Child Adolesc Psychopharmacol*. 2019;29(4):256–267. https://doi.org/10.1089/cap.2018.0136
9. Morgenstern J, Kuerbis A, Shao S, et al. An efficacy trial of adaptive interventions for alcohol use disorder. *J Subst Abuse Treat*. 2021;123:108264. https://doi.org/10.1016/j.jsat.2020.108264
10. Collins LM, Murphy SA, Strecher V. The multiphase optimization strategy (MOST) and the sequential multiple assignment randomized trial (SMART): two novel evaluation methods for developing optimal training programs. *Am J Prev Med*. 2007;32(5, suppl):S112–S118. https://doi.org/10.1016/j.amepre.2007.01.022
11. Lei H, Nahum-Shani I, Lynch K, Oslin D, Murphy SAA. "SMART" design for building individualized treatment sequences. *Annu Rev Clin Psychol*. 2012;8:21–48. https://doi.org/10.1146/annurev-clinpsy-032511-143152
12. Almirall D, Compton SN, Gunlicks-Stoessel M, Duan N, Murphy SA. Designing a pilot sequential multiple assignment randomized trial for developing an adaptive treatment strategy. *Stat Med*. 2012;31(17):1887–1902. https://doi.org/10.1002/sim.4512
13. Kidwell KM, Postow MA, Panageas KS. Sequential, multiple assignment, randomized trial designs in immuno-oncology research. *Clin Cancer Res*. 2018;24(4):730–736. https://doi.org/10.1158/1078-0432.CCR-17-1355
14. Kidwell KM, Hyde LW. Adaptive interventions and SMART designs: application to child behavior research in a community setting. *Am J Eval*. 2016; 37(3):344–363. https://doi.org/10.1177/1098214015617013
15. Almirall D, Nahum-Shani I, Sherwood NE, Murphy SA. Introduction to SMART designs for the development of adaptive interventions: with application to weight loss research. *Transl Behav Med*. 2014;4(3):260–274. https://doi.org/10.1007/s13142-014-0265-0
16. Chakraborty B. Dynamic treatment regimes for managing chronic health conditions: a statistical perspective. *Am J Public Health*. 2011;101(1):40–45. https://doi.org/10.2105/AJPH.2010.198937
17. Dai H, Saccardo S, Han MA, et al. Behavioural nudges increase COVID-19 vaccinations. *Nature*. 2021;597(7876):404–409. https://doi.org/10.1038/s41586-021-03843-2
18. Zhou G. Adaptive interventions for optimizing malaria control: an implementation study protocol for a block-cluster randomized, sequential multiple assignment trial. *Trials*. 2020;21(1):665. https://doi.org/10.1186/s13063-020-04573-y
19. Windsor L, Benoit EM, Pinto R, Sarol J. Optimization of a new adaptive intervention using the SMART design to increase COVID-19 testing among people at high risk in an urban community. *Trials*. 2022;23:310. https://doi.org/10.1186/s13063-022-06216-w
20. Baker TB, Smith SS, Bolt DM, et al. Implementing clinical research using factorial designs: a primer. *Behav Ther*. 2017;48(4):567–580. https://doi.org/10.1016/j.beth.2016.12.005
21. Walton A, Nahum-Shani I, Crosby L, Klasnja P, Murphy S. Optimizing digital integrated care via micro-randomized trials. *Clin Pharmacol Ther*. 2018; 104(1):53–58. https://doi.org/10.1002/cpt.1079
22. Nahum-Shani I, Dziak JJ, Wetter DW. MCMTC: a pragmatic framework for selecting an experimental design to inform the development of digital interventions. *Front Digit Health*. 2022;4: 798025. https://doi.org/10.3389/fdgth.2022.798025
23. Almirall D, Nahum-Shani I, Wang L, Kasari C. Experimental designs for research on adaptive interventions: singly and sequentially randomized trials. In: Collins LM, Kugler KC, eds. *Optimization of Behavioral, Biobehavioral, and Biomedical Interventions: Advanced Topics*. Cham, Switzerland: Springer International; 2018:89–120. https://doi.org/10.1007/978-3-319-91776-4_4
24. Ko JH, Wahed AS. Up-front versus sequential randomizations for inference on adaptive treatment strategies. *Stat Med*. 2012;31(9):812–830. https://doi.org/10.1002/sim.4473
25. Yan X, Matchar DB, Sivapragasam N, Ansah JP, Goel A, Chakraborty B. Sequential multiple assignment randomized trial (SMART) to identify optimal sequences of telemedicine interventions for improving initiation of insulin therapy: a simulation study. *BMC Med Res Methodol*. 2021; 21(1):200. https://doi.org/10.1186/s12874-021-01395-7

26. Yan X, Ghosh P, Chakraborty B. Sample size calculation based on precision for pilot sequential multiple assignment randomized trial (SMART). *Biom J.* 2021;63(2):247–271. https://doi.org/10.1002/bimj.201900364
27. Yan X, Dunne DM, Impey SG, et al. A pilot sequential multiple assignment randomized trial (SMART) protocol for developing an adaptive coaching intervention around a mobile application for athletes to improve carbohydrate periodization behavior. *Contemp Clin Trials Commun.* 2022;26:100899. https://doi.org/10.1016/j.conctc.2022.100899
28. Lambert SD, Grover S, Laizner AM, et al. Adaptive web-based stress management programs among adults with a cardiovascular disease: a pilot sequential multiple assignment randomized trial (SMART). *Patient Educ Couns.* 2022;105(6):1587–1597. https://doi.org/10.1016/j.pec.2021.10.020
29. Oetting AI, Levy JA, Weiss RD, Murphy SA. Statistical methodology for a SMART design in the development of adaptive treatment strategies. In: Shrout P, Keyes K, Ornstein K, eds., *Causality and Psychopathology: Finding the Determinants of Disorders and Their Cures.* New York, NY: Oxford University Press; 2011:179–205. https://doi.org/10.1093/oso/9780199754649.003.0013
30. Ogbagaber SB, Karp J, Wahed AS. Design of sequentially randomized trials for testing adaptive treatment strategies. *Stat Med.* 2016;35(6):840–858. https://doi.org/10.1002/sim.6747
31. Zhong X, Cheng B, Qian M, Cheung YK. A gatekeeping test for selecting adaptive interventions under general designs of sequential multiple assignment randomized trials. *Contemp Clin Trials.* 2019;85:105830. https://doi.org/10.1016/j.cct.2019.105830
32. Zhong T, Wang X, Cheng B, Cheung YK. SMARTAR: sequential multiple assignment randomized trial and adaptive randomization. R Package version 1.1.0. Available at: https://CRAN.R-project.org/package=SMARTAR. Accessed October 28, 2022.
33. Ghosh P, Cheung YK, Chakraborty B. Sample size calculations for clustered SMART designs. In: Kosorok MR, Moodie EEM, eds., *Adaptive Treatment Strategies in Practice.* Philadelphia, PA: Society for Industrial and Applied Mathematics; 2015: 55–70. https://doi.org/10.1137/1.9781611974188.ch5
34. Kidwell KM, Seewald NJ, Tran Q, Kasari C, Almirall D. Design and analysis considerations for comparing dynamic treatment regimens with binary outcomes from sequential multiple assignment randomized trials. *J Appl Stat.* 2018;45(9):1628–1651. https://doi.org/10.1080/02664763.2017.1386773
35. Li Z, Murphy SA. Sample size formulae for two-stage randomized trials with survival outcomes. *Biometrika.* 2011;98(3):503–518. https://doi.org/10.1093/biomet/asr019
36. Seewald NJ, Kidwell KM, Nahum-Shani I, Wu T, McKay JR, Almirall D. Sample size considerations for comparing dynamic treatment regimens in a sequential multiple-assignment randomized trial with a continuous longitudinal outcome. *Stat Methods Med Res.* 2020;29(7):1891–1912. https://doi.org/10.1177/0962280219877520
37. Ghosh P, Yan X, Chakraborty B. A novel approach to assess dynamic treatment regimes embedded in a smart with an ordinal outcome. April 2022. Available at: http://arxiv.org/abs/1808.07287. Accessed June 25, 2022.
38. Quanbeck A, Almirall D, Jacobson N, et al. The balanced opioid initiative: protocol for a clustered, sequential, multiple-assignment randomized trial to construct an adaptive implementation strategy to improve guideline-concordant opioid prescribing in primary care. *Implement Sci.* 2020;15(1):26. https://doi.org/10.1186/s13012-020-00990-4
39. Necamp T, Kilbourne A, Almirall D. Comparing cluster-level dynamic treatment regimens using sequential, multiple assignment, randomized trials: regression estimation and sample size considerations. *Stat Methods Med Res.* 2017; 26(4):1572–1589. https://doi.org/10.1177/0962280217708654
40. Xu J, Bandyopadhyay D, Salehabadi SM, Michalowicz B, Chakraborty B. SMARTp: a SMART design for nonsurgical treatments of chronic periodontitis with spatially referenced and nonrandomly missing skewed outcomes. *Biom J.* 2020;62(2):282–310. https://doi.org/10.1002/bimj.201900027
41. Xu J, Bandyopadhyay D, Azevedo D, Chakraborty B. SMARTp: sample size for SMART designs in non-surgical periodontal trials. R package version 0.1.1. Available at: https://CRAN.R-project.org/package=SMARTp. Accessed October 28, 2022.
42. Ghosh P, Nahum-Shani I, Spring B, Chakraborty B. Noninferiority and equivalence tests in sequential, multiple assignment, randomized trials (SMARTs). *Psychol Methods.* 2020;25(2):182–205. https://doi.org/10.1037/met0000232
43. Artman WJ, Nahum-Shani I, Wu T, Mckay JR, Ertefaie A. Power analysis in a SMART design: sample size estimation for determining the best embedded dynamic treatment regime. *Biostatistics.* 2020;21(3):432–448. https://doi.org/10.1093/biostatistics/kxy064
44. Artman W. Smartsizer: power analysis for a SMART design. R package version 1.0.3. Available at: https://CRAN.R-project.org/package=smartsizer. Accessed October 28, 2022.
45. Artman WJ, Johnson BA, Lynch KG, McKay JR, Ertefaie A. Bayesian set of best dynamic treatment regimes: construction and sample size calculation for SMARTs with binary outcomes. *Stat Med.* 2022;41(9):1688–1708. https://doi.org/10.1002/sim.9323
46. Artman W. SMARTbayesR: Bayesian set of best dynamic treatment regimes and sample size in SMARTs for binary outcomes. R package version 2.0.0. Available at: https://CRAN.R-project.org/package=SMARTbayesR. Accessed October 28, 2022.
47. Rose EJ, Laber EB, Davidian M, Tsiatis AA, Zhao YQ, Kosorok MR. Sample size calculations for SMARTs. June 2019. Available at: http://arxiv.org/abs/1906.06646. Accessed June 24, 2022.
48. Kidwell KM, Wahed AS. Weighted log-rank statistic to compare shared-path adaptive treatment strategies. *Biostatistics.* 2013;14(2):299–312. https://doi.org/10.1093/biostatistics/kxs042
49. Jiang R, Lu W, Song R, Davidian M. On estimation of optimal treatment regimes for maximizing t-year survival probability. *J R Stat Soc Series B Stat Methodol.* 2017;79(4):1165–1185. https://doi.org/10.1111/rssb.12201
50. Chao YC, Tran Q, Tsodikov A, Kidwell KM. Joint modeling and multiple comparisons with the best of data from a SMART with survival outcomes. *Biostatistics.* 2022;23(1):294–313. https://doi.org/10.1093/biostatistics/kxaa025
51. Orellana L, Rotnitzky A, Robins JM. Dynamic regime marginal structural mean models for estimation of optimal dynamic treatment regimes. Part I: main content. *Int J Biostat.* 2010;6(2):8. https://doi.org/10.2202/1557-4679.1200
52. Nahum-Shani I, Qian M, Almirall D, et al. Experimental design and primary data analysis methods for comparing adaptive interventions. *Psychol Methods.* 2012;17(4):457–477. https://doi.org/10.1037/a0029372
53. Lu X, Nahum-Shani I, Kasari C, et al. Comparing dynamic treatment regimes using repeated-measures outcomes: modeling considerations in SMART studies. *Stat Med.* 2016;35(10):1595–1615. https://doi.org/10.1002/sim.6819
54. Kasari C, Kaiser A, Goods K, et al. Communication interventions for minimally verbal children with autism: a sequential multiple assignment randomized trial. *J Am Acad Child Adolesc Psychiatry.* 2014;53(6):635–646. https://doi.org/10.1016/j.jaac.2014.01.019
55. Pelham WE, Fabiano GA, Waxmonsky JG, et al. Treatment sequencing for childhood ADHD: a multiple-randomization study of adaptive medication and behavioral interventions. *J Clin Child Adolesc Psychol.* 2016;45(4):396–415. https://doi.org/10.1080/15374416.2015.1105138
56. Nahum-Shani I, Qian M, Almirall D, et al. Q-learning: a data analysis method for constructing adaptive interventions. *Psychol Methods.* 2012;17(4):478–494. https://doi.org/10.1037/a0029373
57. Zhao Y, Zeng D, Rush AJ, Kosorok MR. Estimating individualized treatment rules using outcome weighted learning. *J Am Stat Assoc.* 2012; 107(449):1106–1118. https://doi.org/10.1080/01621459.2012.695674
58. Laber EB, Zhao YQ. Tree-based methods for individualized treatment regimes. *Biometrika.* 2015; 102(3):501–514. https://doi.org/10.1093/biomet/asv028
59. Zhou X, Mayer-Hamblett N, Khan U, Kosorok MR. Residual weighted learning for estimating individualized treatment rules. *J Am Stat Assoc.* 2017; 112(517):169–187. https://doi.org/10.1080/01621459.2015.1093947
60. Tang X, Melguizo M. DTR: an R package for estimation and comparison of survival outcomes of dynamic treatment regimes. *J Stat Softw.* 2015; 65(7):1–28. https://doi.org/10.18637/jss.v065.i07
61. Chen Y, Liu Y, Zeng D, Wang Y. DTRlearn2: statistical learning methods for optimizing dynamic treatment regimes. R package version 1.1. Available at: https://CRAN.R-project.org/package=DTRlearn2. Accessed October 28, 2022.
62. Wallace M, Moodie EEM, Stephens DA, Schulz GS, Rreg JDT. DTR estimation and inference via G-estimation, dynamic WOLS, Q-Learning, and dynamic weighted survival modeling (DWSurv). R package version 1.7. Available at: https://CRAN.R-project.org/package=DTRreg. Accessed October 28, 2022.
63. Holloway ST, Laber EB, Linn KA, Zhang B, Davidian M, Tsiatis AA. DynTxRegime: methods for estimating optimal dynamic treatment regimes. R package version 4.10. Available at: https://CRAN.R-project.org/package=DynTxRegime. Accessed October 28, 2022.
64. Liu Y, Wang Y, Zeng D. Sequential multiple assignment randomization trials with enrichment design. *Biometrics.* 2017;73(2):378–390. https://doi.org/10.1111/biom.12576

65. Shortreed SM, Laber E, Scott Stroup T, Pineau J, Murphy SA. A multiple imputation strategy for sequential multiple assignment randomized trials. *Stat Med.* 2014;33(24):4202–4214. https://doi.org/10.1002/sim.6223
66. Matrajt L, Eaton J, Leung T, Brown ER. Vaccine optimization for COVID-19: who to vaccinate first? *Sci Adv.* 2021;7(6):eabf1374. https://doi.org/10.1126/sciadv.abf1374
67. Morciano A, Moerbeek M. Optimal allocation to treatments in a sequential multiple assignment randomized trial. *Stat Methods Med Res.* 2021;30(11):2471–2484. https://doi.org/10.1177/09622802211037066
68. Xu Y, Greene TH, Bress AP, et al. Estimating the optimal individualized treatment rule from a cost-effectiveness perspective. *Biometrics.* 2022;78(1):337–351. https://doi.org/10.1111/biom.13406
69. Wu L, Wang J, Wahed AS. Interim monitoring in sequential multiple assignment randomized trials. *Biometrics.* 2021; Epub ahead of print. https://doi.org/10.1111/biom.13562.
70. Cheung YK, Chakraborty B, Davidson KW. Sequential multiple assignment randomized trial (SMART) with adaptive randomization for quality improvement in depression treatment program. *Biometrics.* 2015;71(2):450–459. https://doi.org/10.1111/biom.12258
71. Wang J, Wu L, Wahed AS. Adaptive randomization in a two-stage sequential multiple assignment randomized trial. *Biostatistics.* 2022;23(4):1182–1199. https://doi.org/10.1093/biostatistics/kxab020
72. Ruppert AS, Yin J, Davidian M, et al. Application of a sequential multiple assignment randomized trial (SMART) design in older patients with chronic lymphocytic leukemia. *Ann Oncol.* 2019;30(4):542–550. https://doi.org/10.1093/annonc/mdz053
73. National Library of Medicine. Randomised evaluation of COVID-19 therapy (RECOVERY). May 2021. Available at: https://clinicaltrials.gov/ct2/show/NCT04381936. Accessed September 13, 2022.

Microrandomized Trials: Developing Just-in-Time Adaptive Interventions for Better Public Health

Xueqing Liu, MSc, Nina Deliu, PhD, and Bibhas Chakraborty, PhD

See also Vaughan, p. 35, Seewald, p. 37, Bauer et al., p. 40, and Wang and Chakraborty, p. 49.

Just-in-time adaptive interventions (JITAIs) represent an intervention design that adapts the provision and type of support over time to an individual's changing status and contexts, intending to deliver the right support on the right occasion. As a novel strategy for delivering mobile health interventions, JITAIs have the potential to improve access to quality care in underserved communities and, thus, alleviate health disparities, a significant public health concern.

Valid experimental designs and analysis methods are required to inform the development of JITAIs. Here, we briefly review the cutting-edge design of microrandomized trials (MRTs), covering both the classical MRT design and its outcome-adaptive counterpart.

Associated statistical challenges related to the design and analysis of MRTs are also discussed. Two case studies are provided to illustrate the aforementioned concepts and designs throughout the article. We hope our work leads to better design and application of JITAIs, advancing public health research and practice. (*Am J Public Health*. 2023;113(1):60–69. https://doi.org/10.2105/AJPH.2022.307150)

AJPH January 2023, Vol 113, No. 1

Just-in-time adaptive interventions (JITAIs), also known as dynamic tailoring,[1] ecological momentary interventions,[2] and intelligent real-time therapy,[3] represent an intervention design that adjusts the provision and type of support over time to deal with an individual's changing status and contexts, which intend to deliver the most appropriate support on the right occasion.[4,5] The microrandomized trial (MRT) design has been proposed in recent years as a novel experimental design to construct evidence-based JITAIs. According to this design, participants are sequentially randomized to different intervention options (e.g., whether to send a text message).[6,7] Briefly speaking, JITAIs involve strategies that determine when to intervene and which intervention to provide, while MRTs focus on the optimization of such strategies by selecting and optimizing intervention components for use in a JITAI.

There are 2 key concepts that distinguish JITAIs from standard interventions: just-in-time and adaptive.[5] By just-in-time, JITAIs intend to intervene only when needed to alleviate the intervention fatigue and low engagement problems. On the other hand, adaptive refers to the strategy employed by the intervention design to determine which intervention to provide and when to intervene according to the user's ongoing information. To capture the right timings, JITAIs require continuous monitoring of the user's internal state and contexts, typically via sensors in mobile phones or wearable devices. As a result, delivering just-in-time interventions face to face is not feasible in practice; JITAIs heavily rely on the use of mobile health (mHealth) technologies.[5]

The JITAI in mHealth has the potential to enhance health care and reduce health disparities,[8,9] benefiting various domains of public health research and practice. The MRT has been deliberately introduced to assist with developing these interventions, which can provide information about the dynamics of the best intervention beyond theories and directly inform the construction of JITAIs.[6] Nevertheless, JITAIs and MRTs have not yet been widely adopted in public health, partly because of the unfamiliarity with the concepts, designs, and analysis methods.

With this article, we aim to introduce key ideas in JITAIs, especially focusing on the novel experimental design of MRTs, covering both classical MRT design and its outcome-adaptive counterpart. We discuss the main characteristics of JITAIs along with their potential in public health by relating to 2 mHealth studies with embedded MRT design. We also highlight statistical considerations when designing and analyzing MRTs.

OVERVIEW OF INTERVENTION AND TRIAL DESIGN

The JITAI is an intervention design aiming to deliver adaptive and personalized support only at the time when needed.[4,5] A JITAI consists of 6 key components: decision points, tailoring variables, intervention options, decision rules, proximal outcomes, and distal outcomes.[5] The specific definitions are summarized in Box 1. An intervention option is selected at each decision point based on the values of tailoring variables via a predefined decision rule. The intervention is expected to achieve the distal outcomes by directly impacting the proximal outcomes.

On the other hand, the MRT is an experimental design that provides evidence for building JITAIs. It involves the serial randomization of individuals to different intervention options at each decision point.[5] In general, they can answer several essential research questions arising from the construction of JITAIs:[6,7]

1. Which intervention will have an impact on the proximal outcomes (proximal effects)?
2. What baseline or time-varying covariates will moderate the proximal effects (moderating effects)?
3. How will the proximal effects change over time?
4. When and how frequently should the intervention be delivered?

In what follows, we will illustrate the MRT design and how it connects to the construction of JITAIs by describing 2 mHealth studies: StayWell at Home and Diabetes and Mental Health Adaptive Notification Tracking and Evaluation (DIAMANTE).

Case Studies

StayWell at Home. The StayWell at Home trial examined the effect of a 60-day text messaging intervention that intended to help individuals manage their depression and anxiety during the COVID-19 pandemic.[10] This MRT consisted of adults aged 18 years or older who had a functioning mobile phone and spoke English or Spanish. Figure 1 shows the study design of StayWell at Home.

The distal outcome was the management of depression and anxiety during COVID-19 social distancing. The proximal outcome was a daily mood rating in the following 3 hours after receiving the message, an intermediate measure of the distal outcome that captures short-term progress toward better management of depression and anxiety. The intervention was supportive text messages, half related to behavioral activation and half about coping skills. Many contextual variables were also collected, including time-independent variables such as demographics and questionnaire data and time-varying variables such as study day and yesterday's mood rating. The decision point was chosen among 3 timeframes, including 9 AM to 12 PM, 12 PM to 3 PM, and 3 PM to 6 PM.

In this design, all participants received uniform random messages. The randomization probability for each message category (behavioral

BOX 1— Definitions and Examples of Just-in-Time Adaptive Intervention (JITAI) Components

Components	Definitions	Examples (DIAMANTE)
Decision points	Time points or steps at which an intervention decision is made	Once per day (selected within 4 timeframes by an RL algorithm)
Tailoring variables	Individual information and real-world external context	Demographics, health status, and other baseline information; day of study; number of steps walked yesterday; days since each message type was sent
Intervention options	Various types or amounts of support	Motivational messages (4 categories), feedback messages (5 categories)
Decision rules	The strategy that specifies which intervention option to provide at each decision point according to the tailoring information	Optimized by an RL algorithm (linear Thompson sampling)
Proximal outcomes	The short-term goals the intervention options are intended to achieve, which can be mediators or intermediate measures of the distal outcome	Change in daily step counts
Distal outcomes	The ultimate goals of the JITAI, usually a primary clinical outcome	Diabetes and depression

Note. DIAMANTE = Diabetes and Mental Health Adaptive Notification Tracking and Evaluation; RL = reinforcement learning.

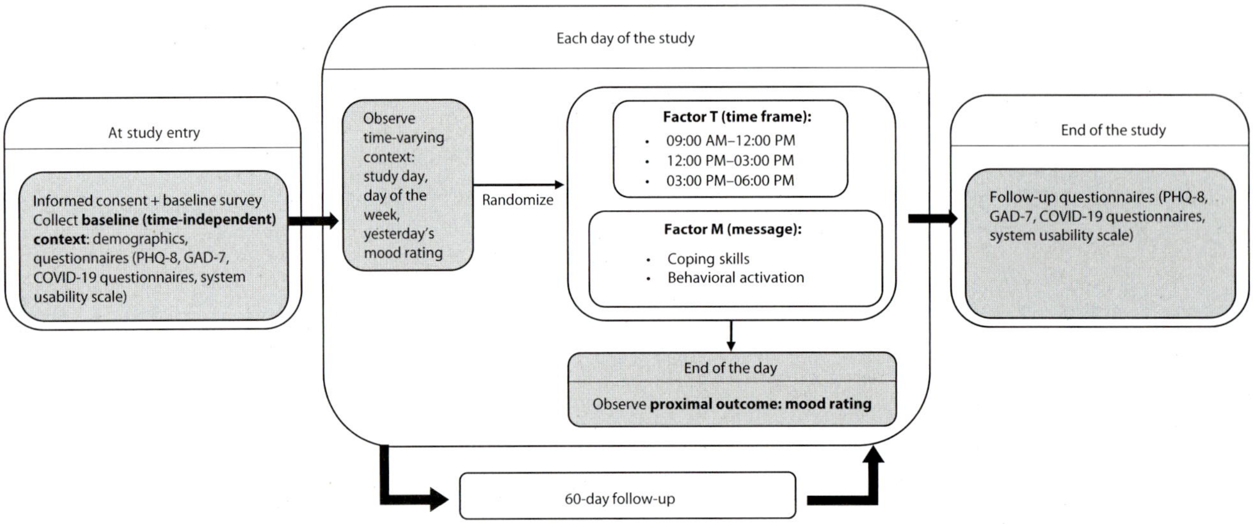

FIGURE 1— **Schematic of the Microrandomized Trial (MRT) Design of the StayWell at Home Study**

Note. GAD-7 = 7-item Generalized Anxiety Disorder Questionnaire; PHQ-8 = 8-item Patient Health Questionnaire.

activation vs coping skill) was 0.5, and the probability for each of the 3 timeframes was 0.33. The collected data allowed for pre–post analysis (i.e., the difference in depression and anxiety levels before and after receiving StayWell messages and the differential effects on mood ratings for the 2 categories of messages and different timings). The pre–post analysis has already been published,[11] while the analysis of MRT data is still underway.

Diabetes and Mental Health Adaptive Notification Tracking and Evaluation. The DIAMANTE trial aimed to evaluate the effect of a text-messaging smartphone application targeting diabetes and depression management through an intermediate outcome representing physical activity.[12] This 6-month MRT study consisted of patients aged 18 to 75 years being treated at the Zuckerberg San Francisco General Hospital who had been diagnosed with diabetes and documented depressive symptoms. Figure 2 presents an overview of the design of this study.

The distal outcome was the improvement of clinical outcomes for comorbid diabetes and depression among low-income, low–health literacy, and ethnic minority individuals. Because lack of physical activity is an overlapping risk factor for these diseases, the embedded intervention was focused on improving an easy-to-measure proximal outcome (i.e., changes in daily step count). A multicomponent intervention consisting of motivational messages (4 categories) and feedback messages (5 categories) were adopted in DIAMANTE. Many contextual variables were collected during the study, including time-independent variables such as demographics, mobile technology familiarity, and other engagement measures, and time-varying variables such as study day and day of the week. The decision point was determined either by uniform randomization or some algorithm among 4 time-frames—that is, 9 AM to 11:30 AM, 11:30 AM to 2 PM, 2 PM to 4:30 PM, and 4:30 PM to 7 PM.

At the macro level, this study is a randomized controlled trial with 3 groups, including a uniform random messaging group, an outcome-adaptive messaging group operationalized through reinforcement learning (RL), and a control group. Participants in the control group received no intervention during the study. With 3 groups, it enables the comparison of adaptive messaging to uniform messaging and no intervention. In the initial 2 weeks, uniform randomization was employed in both the uniform random messaging group and the adaptive messaging group to speed up algorithm learning. After that, the uniform random messaging group used a classical MRT design. Patients received up to 2 randomly selected messages per day within 4 randomly selected timeframes. For the adaptive messaging group, the message categories and timing were chosen by a reinforcement learning algorithm (i.e., linear Thompson sampling).[13] During the conduct of the trial, a JITAI is constructed concurrently, and its characteristics are summarized in Box 1. Data collection for this MRT is currently under way.

Key Design Elements

As an experimental design for empirically informing the construction of

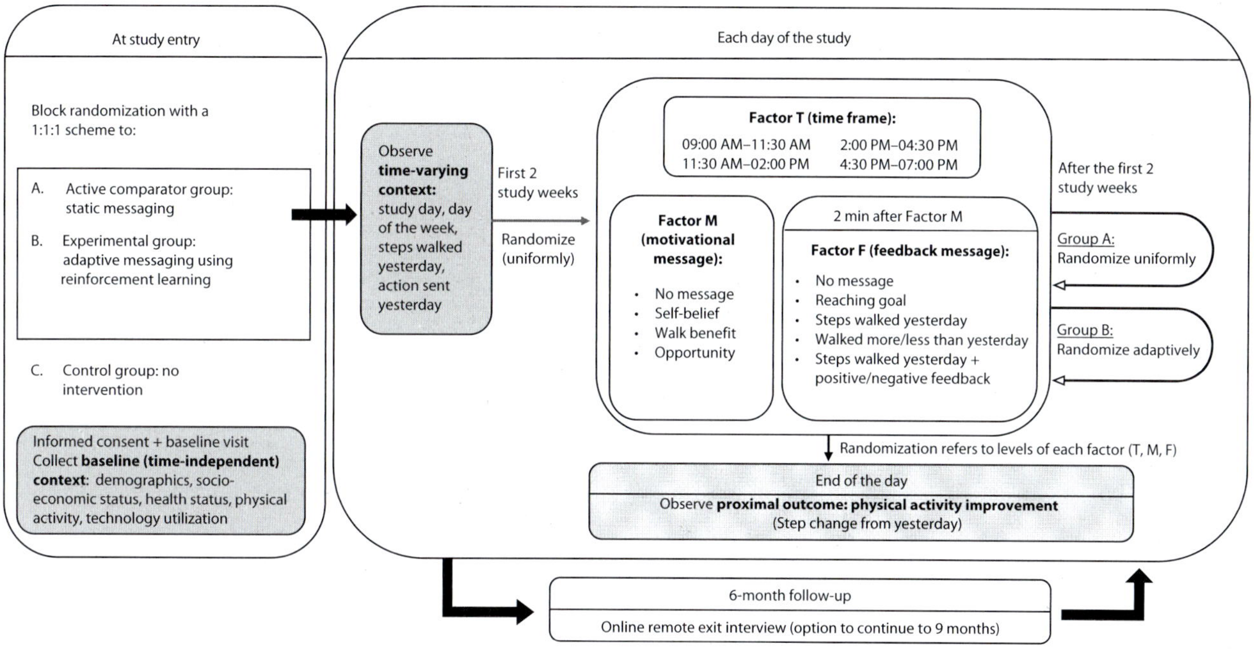

FIGURE 2— **Schematic of the Microrandomized Trial (MRT) Design of the DIAMANTE Study**

Note. DIAMANTE = Diabetes and Mental Health Adaptive Notification Tracking and Evaluation.

JITAIs, the design elements of an MRT study should be tightly connected with JITAI components. The intervention and tailoring variables included in a JITAI are usually supported by theoretical and empirical evidence. An intervention may consist of several components, and each of them may have multiple options. MRTs can be used to assess the proximal effects of 1 or more components simultaneously (e.g., motivational and feedback messages in DIAMANTE). During an MRT, it is essential to collect potential tailoring variables, including individual information and external contexts. These variables can serve as an indicator of individual availability.[14] In the HeartSteps I study, if a participant was driving or already walking, it was considered inappropriate to deliver an activity suggestion, and, thus, the participant was considered unavailable.[15] Potential moderation effects can also be investigated by collecting these variables.

The decision points are determined by the frequency of meaningful changes in the tailoring variables (suggested by empirical evidence and theories), as well as the associated assessment burden.[5] They might occur (1) at a prespecified time interval, (2) at specific times of day or days of week, or (3) following random prompts.[5] MRTs can also provide useful information regarding the selection of decision points. In both DIAMANTE and StayWell at Home, meaningful changes in an individual's context were expected to occur daily. As a result, there was 1 decision point per day. Furthermore, timeframes were treated as an experimental factor to examine the differential intervention effects, which can address the question of when to intervene each day.

At each decision point, participants are randomized to various options of an intervention component—for example, different categories of text messages in DIAMANTE and StayWell at Home, based on predetermined probabilities. These interventions are intended to have an impact on a distal outcome (e.g., diabetes or depression) by affecting an easy-to-measure proximal outcome (e.g., daily step count). Proximal outcomes are often specified as mediators of the distal outcome.[5] For example, ample evidence suggests that lack of physical activity is a risk factor for diabetes and depression. If the target distal outcome is comorbid diabetes and depression, physical activity would be a natural choice for the proximal outcome.[12]

In some cases, the distal outcomes are sustainable behavior change with limited knowledge of corresponding mediators; hence, proximal outcomes can also be short-term measures of the distal outcome.[5] For example, daily mood rating is an intermediate measure of depression and anxiety and can be an appropriate proximal outcome.[10] Note that the distal outcome can be affected by the intervention through multiple causal pathways, leading to a multivariate proximal outcome at each decision time in practice.[5] For example, the proximal outcomes in DIAMANTE and StayWell at Home concern the mechanism lying behind the clinical condition. However, the engagement with intervention may also affect the distal outcome and can be targeted by a JITAI.[5]

During an MRT, each participant may be randomized hundreds or even thousands of times (e.g., 180 times in DIAMANTE and 60 times in StayWell at Home). Randomization permits valid estimation of the intervention's time-varying proximal effects, as it balances unobserved covariates between the intervention options. An important design element of an MRT is randomization probability—that is, the probability of assigning participants to each option of the intervention component. They are motivated by both scientific and practical considerations. For example, assigning higher probabilities to less-demanding options may reduce participant burden. According to whether the randomization probabilities are updated to prioritize the intervention appearing to be optimal, MRTs can be further categorized as classical (e.g., in StayWell at Home) or outcome-adaptive (e.g., in DIAMANTE).[16] We will illustrate these 2 versions of MRTs in the next section.

Classical Vs Outcome-Adaptive Trial Design

Within the classical MRTs, participants are repeatedly randomized to different intervention options according to a fixed time-invariant scheme (i.e., a scheme wherein the probabilities of being allocated to each intervention option remain uniform over time) or a time-varying allocation strategy, (i.e., a strategy wherein the randomization probabilities depend on the individual's previous observations).[17,18] Specifically, the latter seeks to avoid excess burden by constraining the number of interventions per day and to spread the interventions uniformly across different strata of decision points (e.g., stressed minutes or nonstressed minutes).[19]

However, classical MRTs focus on post–data-collection JITAI optimization (i.e., data analysis is conducted at the end of the trial [known as "offline" learning in the computer science literature]). Such classical MRTs share similarities with the traditional fixed design (with fixed randomization probabilities) or the biased coin design (with time-varying randomization probabilities) of randomized clinical trials,[20] where interventions appearing to be desirable for users (i.e., showing better effectiveness) cannot be prioritized during the trial. The goal is to collect high-quality data that may inform practices for future patients, while participants of the current trial cannot benefit from the new findings.[16]

For outcome-adaptive MRTs, the randomization probabilities are adaptively changed in favor of intervention options with superior performance or the highest expected proximal outcome.[16] An essential feature of outcome-adaptive MRTs is that the randomization probabilities are continually adjusted so that the user is assigned to an intervention appearing to be optimal with a higher chance. The outcome-adaptive MRT involves a number of interim analyses during the trial: at every decision point, the design algorithm, usually a reinforcement learning algorithm, selects an intervention option based on historical proximal outcomes and current context, enabling the timely delivery of proper support when needed (known as online learning in the computer science literature). This process leads to an online version of JITAI, which is certainly not the case with classical MRTs.

The outcome-adaptive MRT design is more ethical and efficient when compared with its classical counterpart. First, it can benefit current participants as the intervention delivery is continually optimized to their current context,[16] intending to maximize the cumulative proximal outcomes. The design algorithm can also uncover effective predictors of the right timings when users are more likely to benefit from support and can monitor changes in these predictors, triggering appropriate interventions when needed.[16] Furthermore, the outcome-adaptive MRT may save money by avoiding the collection of useless covariates (i.e., covariates not moderating the intervention effects). More importantly, data collected from outcome-adaptive MRTs can also be used for deriving causal effects and informing offline JITAI construction. Both mHealth and reinforcement learning literatures have provided ways for the analysis of MRTs with time-varying randomization probabilities.[21,22]

Despite that, some drawbacks, such as the increase in trial complexity and the statistical inefficiency caused by unequal allocation,[23] raise questions regarding the use of outcome-adaptive MRTs. As a result, careful considerations should be given to the adoption of outcome-adaptive MRTs, especially to ethical issues (e.g., whether the current participants are in urgent need of interventions) and budget constraints (e.g., balancing between the increased human resources because of trial complexity and the cost reduction during the data collection procedure).

POTENTIALS IN PUBLIC HEALTH

As a plausible substitute for face-to-face interactions, JITAIs in mHealth might assist with enhancing health care and reducing health disparities caused by inequities in health care systems, especially in underserved communities.[8,9] First, the relative cost and scalability of these interventions allow for faster delivery of quality care, particularly critical in emergencies. During the COVID-19 pandemic, there has been a surge in interest and use of mHealth to meet the increasing demands of health care. With physical distancing restrictions and a lack of in-person care, mHealth has the potential to improve access to mental health care[24,25] and enable self-management.[26] For example, participants who received the StayWell text messaging intervention showed improved depression and anxiety symptoms after the study,[11] indicating that such mHealth interventions are beneficial.

Second, the high uptake of mobile technologies among minority and low-income patients has the potential to improve the health care of populations with limited access to traditional health care resources.[27] For example, the DIAMANTE study focused on low-income, low–health literacy, and ethnic minority individuals. These populations may experience higher prevalence and worse outcomes for both diabetes and depression, and, at the same time, they may lack access to health care. Because of the demonstrated effectiveness of DIAMANTE messages,[28] deploying these mHealth interventions can potentially decrease disparities in health care by reaching vulnerable populations.

More importantly, JITAIs have a distinct advantage in capturing the exact moment of users' needs and providing just-in-time support only when it is more likely to benefit the user. As a result, JITAIs may alleviate the practical issues of low engagement and declining effectiveness over time faced by many conventional mHealth interventions, which are delivered uniformly to users without taking into account the contexts and individual information. For these reasons, JITAIs are increasingly being used in various public health domains, including physical activity maintenance,[29] mental health management,[30] weight loss,[31] and smoking cessation.[32] The effectiveness of JITAIs on various health outcomes has been demonstrated in empirical studies.[33] In general, JITAIs hold enormous potential in public health research and practice.

STATISTICAL CHALLENGES FOR MICRORANDOMIZED TRIALS

In this section, we will describe several vital statistical considerations in the design and analysis of MRTs. When designing an MRT, sample size calculation is crucial, while for an outcome-adaptive MRT, the online "adaptive algorithm" for updating the randomization probabilities adds an additional layer of complexity. In what follows, we will briefly review existing methods related to the preceding issues. Other significant challenges are also summarized.

Sample Size Calculations

When calculating the sample size, it is necessary to specify a primary research question out of all questions of interest. In an MRT study, the primary research question is typically the time-varying effects of an intervention component on the proximal outcome, and sample size calculations are performed to ensure an adequate power to detect statistically significant effects. For example, in StayWell at Home, the primary aim was to investigate whether the type of text messages would affect participants' moods. To facilitate MRT design, Liao et al.[34] proposed an approach to determine the sample size for continuous outcomes by modifying sample size formulas originally developed in the context of generalized estimating equations. Seewald et al.[35] developed an online sample size calculator to help domain scientists implement this method. The calculator for binary outcomes can be accessed via https://tqian.shinyapps.io/mrt_ss_binary, while the methodology article has not yet been published online. In addition, Dempsey et al.[17] developed a stratified MRT and provided a sample size formula, and Xu et al.[36] proposed a flexible MRT design allowing for the addition of intervention options during the study and derived corresponding sample size estimators. Box 2 presents information on the sample size calculation methods and software. Nonetheless, other open questions still warrant further research in the design of MRTs, such as the sample size formula for MRTs with count (e.g., number of cigarettes, number of active minutes) or ordinal (e.g., mood rating on a scale of 1–9) proximal outcomes, which are commonly seen in practice.

Randomization Probability Updates

In outcome-adaptive MRTs, the randomization probabilities are continuously changed in favor of better-performing interventions (i.e., the intervention option that can lead to a higher proximal outcome), allowing the optimization of

BOX 2— Summary of Statistical Methods for Sample Size Calculations and Data Analysis in Microrandomized Trials

Method	Outcome Type	Functionality	Software
Sample size calculations			
Liao et al.[34]	Continuous	Sample size calculators for MRTs detecting the proximal effects	R shiny app (MRT-SS-Continuous; https://statisticalreinforcementlearninglab.shinyapps.io/mrt_ss_continuous)
Qian et al.[14]	Binary	Sample size calculators for MRTs detecting the proximal effects	R shiny app (MRT-SS-Binary; https://tqian.shinyapps.io/mrt_ss_binary/)
Dempsey et al.[17]	Continuous	Sample size calculators for stratified MRTs detecting the nested proximal effects	R code (https://github.com/wdempsey/stratified_mrt)
Xu et al.[36]	Continuous	Sample size calculators for flexible MRTs (which allows for flexible addition of intervention options) detecting the proximal effects	R shiny app (FlexiMRT-SS; https://kennyxu.shinyapps.io/FlexiMRT-SS)
Data analysis			
Boruvka et al.[21]	Continuous	Estimating causal excursion effect (moderation) of a time-varying component on a time-varying outcome	R (geepack; https://cran.r-project.org/web/packages/geepack/index.html/ geeM; https://cran.r-project.org/web/packages/geeM/geeM.pdf), SAS (PROC GEE; https://documentation.sas.com/doc/en/pgmsascdc/9.4_3.4/statug/statug_gee_syntax01.htm), Stata (xtgee; https://www.stata.com/features/overview/generalized-estimating-equations/) R code for small sample correction; https://github.com/StatisticalReinforcementLearningLab/HeartstepsV1Code/blob/master/xgeepack.R
Qian et al.[37]	Binary	Estimating causal excursion effect (moderation) of a time-varying component on a time-varying outcome	R code (https://github.com/tqian/binary-outcome-mrt)
Shi et al.[38]	Continuous	Estimating causal excursion effect (moderation) of a time-varying component on a time-varying outcome under potential cluster-level treatment effect and interference	R code (https://github.com/Herashi/MRT-mHealthModeration)
Li and Wager[39]	Binary	Estimating various causal estimands (short-term and long-term direct effect, long-term total effect) under cross-unit interference	NA

Note. MRT = microrandomized trial; NA = not available.

online JITAIs. Reinforcement learning provides an ideal framework for solving such sequential decision-making problems:[40] an agent continuously interacts with a stochastic environment, or the context, and learns how to make better actions or interventions to maximize the cumulative feedback or proximal outcome over time.

Currently, most methods for constructing JITAIs online within the outcome-adaptive MRT fall in a subcategory of RL (i.e., contextual multiarmed bandits).[41] Various algorithms have been proposed for contextual multiarmed bandits, making different assumptions about the data-generating process.[41,42] In particular, Thompson sampling has demonstrated not only valid theoretical performance guarantees but also strong empirical performance.[43,44] Because of these advantages, as well as its randomized exploration nature, Thompson sampling has been adopted in the DIAMANTE[12] study and the HeartSteps II study.[45] In addition, other reinforcement learning methods have been employed in mHealth studies. We refer readers to Deliu et al.[42] and Tewari and Murphy[41] for comprehensive reviews of existing RL approaches for developing JITAIs, and to Trella et al.[46] and Figueroa et al.[47] for guidelines regarding the design of online RL algorithms for mHealth interventions.

Data Analysis

Analyzing MRT data and deriving causal effects are critical steps for constructing efficacious JITAIs. Because MRT data include time-varying interventions and endogenous covariates (i.e., depends on previous interventions or outcomes), standard methods for longitudinal data, including generalized estimating equations and mixed effect approaches, can lead to inconsistent estimates of causal effects.[48]

A weighted and centered least squares (WCLS) estimation procedure has been proposed to obtain unbiased estimates of the causal excursion effects of time-varying components on a time-varying continuous outcome.[21] With some modifications, the WCLS estimator and its standard error can be derived using standard software for generalized estimating equations,[6,21] such as geepack[49] in R (R Foundation for Statistical Computing, Vienna, Austria) and PROC GEE in SAS (SAS Institute, Cary, NC). This approach can also be generalized to the setting where the randomization probabilities may change over time.[21]

Because the WCLS approach is limited to continuous proximal outcomes, Qian et al.[37] proposed a semiparametric estimator of the causal excursion effect in MRTs with binary proximal outcomes. Furthermore, Shi et al.[38] developed a general inferential approach for the causal excursion effect with continuous outcome under potential cluster-level treatment effect and interference. Li and Wager[39] provided estimation strategies for various causal estimands (i.e., the short-term and long-term direct effect) and the long-term total effect, with a binary outcome under cross-unit interference. See Box 2 for a summary of these methods, as well as the available software. Despite that, specific methods for other data types, such as ordinal or count outcomes, are still not well-developed, as is the case with sample size calculation.

Variable Selection

Within JITAIs, the content and delivery of interventions are tailored to an individual's ongoing information and external context. Hence, it is necessary to collect all relevant contextual variables and assess the moderation effects of each variable. If there is a large number of potential moderators, we need to conduct moderation analyses using the WCLS approach many times, which can be inconvenient and burdensome. For example, the DIAMANTE study has a high number of baseline and time-varying covariates, which may also interact with the interventions. Although Seewald et al.[50] recommended prespecifying the relative "priority" of each variable, in practice, scientists may not have a priori knowledge about these variables. Therefore, how best to select a subset of variables for subsequent moderation analyses remains unresolved.

Missing Data

In the pilot study of DIAMANTE,[28] there were 670 days with missing steps and 3 participants with 2 or fewer days of step data. A critical issue with analyzing MRT data is how to handle these missing data, as missingness may lead to selection bias in subsequent causal inference.[51] However, there is no comprehensive discussion of missing data issues in MRT. In general, 3 methods to handle missing data have been used in MRT studies: complete-case data analysis,[28,52] single imputation,[15] and multiple imputation.[53] In practice, the choice of method should depend on the missingness mechanisms, which can be identified by collecting reasons for missing data during the study.[50] Nevertheless, no matter which method is adopted in the main analysis, sensitivity analysis is recommended to assess the robustness of the findings, especially when data are not missing at random.[54]

CONCLUSION

In this review, we have summarized the general framework of the JITAI emerging in mHealth, as well as the key concepts, design considerations, and statistical challenges of a novel experimental design, MRT, that can empirically inform JITAIs by assessing the proximal effects and moderation effects. In particular, MRTs can be categorized as classical or outcome-adaptive according to whether the randomization probabilities are adaptively updated in favor of the optimal intervention. When designing outcome-adaptive MRTs, researchers need to choose an appropriate reinforcement learning algorithm for updating these probabilities in addition to the sample size considerations. Nonetheless, there are still some challenges concerning designing and analyzing MRT studies—for example, analysis methods for other types of proximal outcomes, variable selection, and missing data.

With this review, we have sought to introduce the intervention design (JITAI), as well as the cutting-edge experimental design (MRT) of mHealth interventions, to a broad range of readers in the field of public health. We hope our work will lead to greater interest among the public health research community in the uptake of JITAIs and MRT methodologies, ultimately leading to the improvement of human lives. AJPH

ABOUT THE AUTHORS

Xueqing Liu is with the Centre for Quantitative Medicine, Duke-National University of Singapore (NUS) Medical School, Singapore. Nina Deliu is with the Medical Research Council Biostatistics Unit, University of Cambridge, UK, and the Department of Methods and Models for Economics, Territory and Finance, Sapienza University of Rome, Italy. Bibhas Chakraborty is with the Centre for Quantitative Medicine and Program in Health Services and Systems Research, Duke-NUS Medical School, Singapore; the Department of Statistics and Data Science, NUS, Singapore; and the

Department of Biostatistics and Bioinformatics, Duke University, Durham, NC.

CORRESPONDENCE

Correspondence should be sent to Bibhas Chakraborty, PhD, Associate Professor, Centre for Quantitative Medicine, Duke-NUS Medical School, 8 College Rd, Level 6, #06-31, Singapore 169857 (e-mail: bibhas.chakraborty@duke-nus.edu.sg). Reprints can be ordered at https://ajph.org by clicking the "Reprints" link.

PUBLICATION INFORMATION

Full Citation: Liu X, Deliu N, Chakraborty B. Micro-randomized trials: developing just-in-time adaptive interventions for better public health. *Am J Public Health*. 2023;113(1):60–69.

Acceptance Date: October 5, 2022.

DOI: https://doi.org/10.2105/AJPH.2022.307150

CONTRIBUTORS

X. Liu wrote the first draft of the article. B. Chakraborty conceptualized the project and developed the outline and topics to be covered. N. Deliu contributed sections of the article. All authors reviewed and approved the final version of the article.

ACKNOWLEDGMENTS

B. Chakraborty would like to acknowledge research support from the Khoo Bridge Funding Award (Duke-NUS-KBrFA/2021/0040) and the start-up grant from the Duke-NUS Medical School, National University of Singapore.

We wish to acknowledge helpful comments from Roger Vaughan, DrPH, MS.

CONFLICTS OF INTEREST

The authors have no conflicts of interest to declare.

HUMAN PARTICIPANT PROTECTION

No protocol approval was needed for this project because no human participants were involved.

REFERENCES

1. Kennedy CM, Powell J, Payne TH, Ainsworth J, Boyd A, Buchan I. Active assistance technology for health-related behavior change: an interdisciplinary review. *J Med Internet Res*. 2012;14(3):e80. https://doi.org/10.2196/jmir.1893
2. Heron KE, Smyth JM. Ecological momentary interventions: incorporating mobile technology into psychosocial and health behaviour treatments. *Br J Health Psychol*. 2010;15(pt 1):1–39. https://doi.org/10.1348/135910709X466063
3. Kelly J, Gooding P, Pratt D, Ainsworth J, Welford M, Tarrier N. Intelligent real-time therapy: harnessing the power of machine learning to optimise the delivery of momentary cognitive–behavioural interventions. *J Ment Health*. 2012;21(4):404–414. https://doi.org/10.3109/09638237.2011.638001
4. Spruijt-Metz D, Wen CKF, O'Reilly G, et al. Innovations in the use of interactive technology to support weight management. *Curr Obes Rep*. 2015;4(4):510–519. https://doi.org/10.1007/s13679-015-0183-6
5. Nahum-Shani I, Smith SN, Spring BJ, et al. Just-in-time adaptive interventions (JITAIs) in mobile health: key components and design principles for ongoing health behavior support. *Ann Behav Med*. 2018;52(6):446–462. https://doi.org/10.1007/s12160-016-9830-8
6. Klasnja P, Hekler EB, Shiffman S, et al. Micro-randomized trials: an experimental design for developing just-in-time adaptive interventions. *Health Psychology*. 2015;34S:1220–1228. https://doi.org/10.1037/hea0000305
7. Golbus JR, Dempsey W, Jackson EA, Nallamothu BK, Klasnja P. Microrandomized trial design for evaluating just-in-time adaptive interventions through mobile health technologies for cardiovascular disease. *Circ Cardiovasc Qual Outcomes*. 2021;14(2):e006760. https://doi.org/10.1161/CIRCOUTCOMES.120.006760
8. Gonzalez BD. Promise of mobile health technology to reduce disparities in patients with cancer and survivors. *JCO Clin Cancer Inform*. 2018;2(2):1–9. https://doi.org/10.1200/CCI.17.00141
9. Hoque MR, Rahman MS, Nipa NJ, Hasan MR. Mobile health interventions in developing countries: a systematic review. *Health Informatics J*. 2020;26(4):2792–2810. https://doi.org/10.1177/1460458220937102
10. Figueroa CA, Hernandez-Ramos R, Boone CE, et al. A text messaging intervention for coping with social distancing during COVID-19 (StayWell at Home): protocol for a randomized controlled trial. *JMIR Res Protoc*. 2021;10(1):e23592. https://doi.org/10.2196/23592
11. Aguilera A, Hernandez-Ramos R, Haro-Ramos AY, et al. A text messaging intervention (StayWell at Home) to counteract depression and anxiety during COVID-19 social distancing: pre–post study. *JMIR Ment Health*. 2021;8(11):e25298. https://doi.org/10.2196/25298
12. Aguilera A, Figueroa CA, Hernandez-Ramos R, et al. mHealth app using machine learning to increase physical activity in diabetes and depression: clinical trial protocol for the DIAMANTE Study. *BMJ Open*. 2020;10(8):e034723. https://doi.org/10.1136/bmjopen-2019-034723
13. Agrawal S, Goyal N. Thompson sampling for contextual bandits with linear payoffs. *PMLR*. 2013;28(3):127–135. Available at: https://proceedings.mlr.press/v28/agrawal13.html. Accessed October 28, 2022.
14. Qian T, Walton AE, Collins LM, et al. The micro-randomized trial for developing digital interventions: experimental design and data analysis considerations. *Psychol Methods*. 2022; epub ahead of print January 13, 2022. https://doi.org/10.1037/met0000283
15. Klasnja P, Smith S, Seewald NJ, et al. Efficacy of contextually tailored suggestions for physical activity: a micro-randomized optimization trial of HeartSteps. *Ann Behav Med*. 2019;53(6):573–582. https://doi.org/10.1093/abm/kay067
16. Saghafian S, Murphy SA. Innovative health care delivery: the scientific and regulatory challenges in designing mHealth interventions. *NAM Perspectives*. Washington, DC: National Academy of Medicine; 2021. https://doi.org/10.31478/202108b
17. Dempsey W, Liao P, Kumar S, Murphy SA. The stratified micro-randomized trial design: sample size considerations for testing nested causal effects of time-varying treatments. *Ann Appl Stat*. 2020;14(2):661–684. https://doi.org/10.1214/19-AOAS1293
18. Liao P, Dempsey W, Sarker H, et al. Just-in-time but not too much: determining treatment timing in mobile health. *Proc ACM Interact Mob Wearable Ubiquitous Technol*. 2018;2(4):1–21. https://doi.org/10.1145/3287057
19. Battalio SL, Conroy DE, Dempsey W, et al. Sense2Stop: a micro-randomized trial using wearable sensors to optimize a just-in-time-adaptive stress management intervention for smoking relapse prevention. *Contemp Clin Trials*. 2021;109:106534. https://doi.org/10.1016/j.cct.2021.106534
20. Rosenberger WF, Sverdlov O, Hu F. Adaptive randomization for clinical trials. *J Biopharm Stat*. 2012;22(4):719–736. https://doi.org/10.1080/10543406.2012.676535
21. Boruvka A, Almirall D, Witkiewitz K, Murphy SA. Assessing time-varying causal effect moderation in mobile health. *J Am Stat Assoc*. 2018;113(523):1112–1121. https://doi.org/10.1080/01621459.2017.1305274
22. Zhang KW, Janson L, Murphy S. Statistical inference with m-estimators on adaptively collected data. *Adv Neural Inf Process Syst*. 2021;34:7460–7471.
23. Korn EL, Freidlin B. Adaptive clinical trials: advantages and disadvantages of various adaptive design elements. *J Natl Cancer Inst*. 2017;109(6):djx013. https://doi.org/10.1093/jnci/djx013
24. Fedele DA, Cushing CC, Fritz A, Amaro CM, Ortega A. Mobile health interventions for improving health outcomes in youth: a meta-analysis. *JAMA Pediatr*. 2017;171(5):461–469. https://doi.org/10.1001/jamapediatrics.2017.0042
25. Firth J, Torous J, Nicholas J, Carney R, Rosenbaum S, Sarris J. Can smartphone mental health interventions reduce symptoms of anxiety? A meta-analysis of randomized controlled trials. *J Affect Disord*. 2017;218:15–22. https://doi.org/10.1016/j.jad.2017.04.046
26. Sasangohar F, Jones SL, Masud FN, Vahidy FS, Kash BA. Provider burnout and fatigue during the COVID-19 pandemic: lessons learned from a high-volume intensive care unit. *Anesth Analg*. 2020;131(1):106–111. https://doi.org/10.1213/ANE.0000000000004866
27. van Veen T, Binz S, Muminovic M, et al. Potential of mobile health technology to reduce health disparities in underserved communities. *West J Emerg Med*. 2019;20(5):799–802. https://doi.org/10.5811/westjem.2019.6.41911
28. Figueroa CA, Deliu N, Chakraborty B, et al. Daily motivational text messages to promote physical activity in university students: results from a microrandomized trial. *Ann Behav Med*. 2022;56(2):212–218. https://doi.org/10.1093/abm/kaab028
29. Hardeman W, Houghton J, Lane K, Jones A, Naughton F. A systematic review of just-in-time adaptive interventions (JITAIs) to promote physical activity. *Int J Behav Nutr Phys Act*. 2019;16(1):31. https://doi.org/10.1186/s12966-019-0792-7
30. Bidargaddi N, Schrader G, Klasnja P, Licinio J, Murphy S. Designing m-health interventions for precision mental health support. *Transl*

Psychiatry. 2020;10(1):222. https://doi.org/10.1038/s41398-020-00895-2

31. Forman EM, Goldstein SP, Crochiere RJ, et al. Randomized controlled trial of OnTrack, a just-in-time adaptive intervention designed to enhance weight loss. *Transl Behav Med*. 2019;9(6):989–1001. https://doi.org/10.1093/tbm/ibz137
32. Cerrada CJ, Dzubur E, Blackman KCA, Mays V, Shoptaw S, Huh J. Development of a just-in-time adaptive intervention for smoking cessation among Korean American emerging adults. *Int J Behav Med*. 2017;24(5):665–672. https://doi.org/10.1007/s12529-016-9628-x
33. Wang L, Miller LC. Just-in-the-moment adaptive interventions (JITAI): a meta-analytical review. *Health Commun*. 2020;35(12):1531–1544. https://doi.org/10.1080/10410236.2019.1652388
34. Liao P, Klasnja P, Tewari A, Murphy SA. Sample size calculations for micro-randomized trials in mHealth. *Stat Med*. 2016;35(12):1944–1971. https://doi.org/10.1002/sim.6847
35. Seewald NJ, Sun J, Liao P. MRT-SS Calculator: an R shiny application for sample size calculation in micro-randomized trials. Preprint. Posted online August 5, 2020. arXiv. 160900695. https://doi.org/10.48550/arXiv.1609.00695
36. Xu J, Yan X, Figueroa C, Williams JJ, Chakraborty B. Micro-randomized trial with flexible design and sample size considerations. Preprint. Posted online October 21, 2022. arXiv. 220314914. https://doi.org/10.48550/arXiv.2203.14914
37. Qian T, Yoo H, Klasnja P, Almirall D, Murphy SA. Estimating time-varying causal excursion effects in mobile health with binary outcomes. *Biometrika*. 2021;108(3):507–527. https://doi.org/10.1093/biomet/asaa070
38. Shi J, Wu Z, Dempsey W. Assessing time-varying causal effect moderation in the presence of cluster-level treatment effect heterogeneity. Preprint. Posted online December 10, 2021. arXiv. 210201681. https://doi.org/10.48550/arXiv.2102.01681
39. Li S, Wager S. Network interference in micro-randomized trials. Preprint. Posted online February 10, 2022. arXiv:220205356. https://doi.org/10.48550/arXiv.2202.05356
40. Sutton RS, Barto AG. *Reinforcement Learning: An Introduction*. Cambridge, MA: The MIT Press; 2018.
41. Tewari A, Murphy SA. From ads to interventions: contextual bandits in mobile health. In: Rehg J, Murphy S, Kumar S, eds. *Mobile Health*. Cham, Switzerland: Springer; 2017:495–517. https://doi.org/10.1007/978-3-319-51394-2_25
42. Deliu N, Williams JJ, Chakraborty B. Reinforcement learning in modern biostatistics: constructing optimal adaptive interventions. Preprint. Posted online March 4, 2022. arXiv. 220302605. https://doi.org/10.48550/arXiv.2203.02605
43. Chapelle O, Li L. An empirical evaluation of Thompson sampling. *Adv Neural Inf Process Syst*. 2011;24:2249–2257. https://dl.acm.org/doi/abs/10.5555/2986459.2986710
44. Osband I, van Roy B. Why is posterior sampling better than optimism for reinforcement learning? *PMLR*. 2017;70:2701–2710. Available at: https://proceedings.mlr.press/v70/osband17a.html. Accessed October 29, 2022.
45. Spruijt-Metz D, Marlin BM, Pavel M, et al. Advancing behavioral intervention and theory development for mobile health: the HeartSteps II protocol. *Int J Environ Res Public Health*. 2022;19(4):2267. https://doi.org/10.3390/ijerph19042267
46. Trella AL, Zhang KW, Nahum-Shani I, Shetty V, Doshi-Velez F, Murphy SA. Designing reinforcement learning algorithms for digital interventions: pre-implementation guidelines. *Algorithms*. 2022;15(8):255. https://doi.org/10.3390/a15080255
47. Figueroa CA, Aguilera A, Chakraborty B, et al. Adaptive learning algorithms to optimize mobile applications for behavioral health: guidelines for design decisions. *J Am Med Inform Assoc*. 2021;28(6):1225–1234. https://doi.org/10.1093/jamia/ocab001
48. Qian T, Klasnja P, Murphy SA. Linear mixed models with endogenous covariates: modeling sequential treatment effects with application to a mobile health study. *Stat Sci*. 2020;35(3):375–390. https://doi.org/10.1214/19-STS720
49. Højsgaard S, Halekoh U, Yan J. The R package geepack for generalized estimating equations. *J Stat Softw*. 2006;15:1–11. https://doi.org/10.18637/jss.v015.i02
50. Seewald NJ, Smith SN, Lee AJ, Klasnja P, Murphy SA. Practical considerations for data collection and management in mobile health micro-randomized trials. *Stat Biosci*. 2019;11(2):355–370. https://doi.org/10.1007/s12561-018-09228-w
51. Rubin DB. Inference and missing data. *Biometrika*. 1976;63(3):581–592. https://doi.org/10.1093/biomet/63.3.581
52. Nahum-Shani I, Rabbi M, Yap J, et al. Translating strategies for promoting engagement in mobile health: a proof-of-concept microrandomized trial. *Health Psychol*. 2021;40(12):971–987. https://doi.org/10.1037/hea0001101
53. NeCamp T, Sen S, Frank E, et al. Assessing real-time moderation for developing adaptive mobile health interventions for medical interns: micro-randomized trial. *J Med Internet Res*. 2020;22(3):e15033. https://doi.org/10.2196/15033
54. Robins JM, Rotnitzky A, Scharfstein DO. Sensitivity analysis for selection bias and unmeasured confounding in missing data and causal inference models. In: Halloran ME, Berry D. *Statistical Models in Epidemiology, the Environment, and Clinical Trials*. New York, NY: Springer; 2000:1–94. https://doi.org/10.1007/978-1-4612-1284-3_1

Antiracism and Community-Based Participatory Research: Synergies, Challenges, and Opportunities

Paul J. Fleming, PhD, MPH, Lisa Cacari Stone, PhD, MA, MS, Melissa S. Creary, PhD, MPH, Ella Greene-Moton, Barbara A. Israel, DrPH, MPH, Kent D. Key, PhD, MPH, Angela G. Reyes, MPH, Nina Wallerstein, DrPH, MPH, and Amy J. Schulz, PhD, MPH, MSW

Structural racism causes stark health inequities and operates at every level of society, including the academic and governmental entities that support health research and practice. We argue that health research institutions must invest in research that actively disrupts racial hierarchies, with leadership from racially marginalized communities and scholars.

We highlight synergies between antiracist principles and community-based participatory research (CBPR), examine the potential for CBPR to promote antiracist research and praxis, illustrate structural barriers to antiracist CBPR praxis, and offer examples of CBPR actions taken to disrupt structural racism. We make recommendations for the next generation of antiracist CBPR, including modify health research funding to center the priorities of racially marginalized communities, support sustained commitments and accountability to those communities by funders and research institutions, distribute research funds equitably across community and academic institutions, amplify antiracist praxis through translation of research to policy, and adopt institutional practices that support reflection and adaptation of CBPR to align with emergent community priorities and antiracist practices.

A critical application of CBPR principles offers pathways to transforming institutional practices that reproduce and reinforce racial inequities. (*Am J Public Health*. 2023;113(1):70–78. https://doi.org/10.2105/AJPH.2022.307114)

AJPH January 2023, Vol 113, No. 1

For decades, community activists and a small number of health scholars have been calling for health researchers to not just study racism but be actively antiracist and contribute to transforming our inequitable systems.[1,2] Recently, an increasing number of health scholars and mainstream public health institutions (e.g., the Centers for Disease Control and Prevention, the National Institutes of Health [NIH]) have called for more antiracist health research that directly confronts and addresses structural racism in both its process and outcomes.[3–7] For example, the NIH launched the UNITE initiative to "identify and address structural racism within the NIH-supported and the greater scientific community."[3] To fulfill these antiracist ambitions, we need bold leadership and expansion of equitable models that disrupt hierarchies embedded in our health research institutions (e.g., the NIH, major universities, nonprofit organizations). These models need to center community voices and support community–academic partnerships to foster racial justice.

Investing in community-based participatory research (CBPR) approaches offers an opportunity for health research institutions to move closer to antiracist principles. CBPR approaches—distinct from the broader term "community-based" research and only a narrow slice of all health research—often actively seek to disrupt racial hierarchies in how they are conducted (i.e., the process) and in the outcomes they seek to affect (i.e., health equity).[2,8–10] Literature reviews demonstrate that CBPR partnerships can have an important positive impact on health outcomes in marginalized communities,[11–13] but these impacts are constrained and limited by pervasive racial inequities embedded in research and funding institutions.[14–17]

The emancipatory roots that underlie CBPR draw from the epistemic traditions of oppressed communities of color and Indigenous communities across the globe that have sought to facilitate community empowerment and agency.[18] The liberatory foundations of CBPR are anchored in Brazilian educator Paulo Freire's dialogical approach to critical consciousness and the cyclical praxis of reflection and action; in Global South movements to end apartheid (e.g., in South Africa) and build knowledge democracy; and in civil rights movements to end White supremacy in the United States.[12,18–20]

Building on these historical roots, since the 1990s a growing community of health scholars has partnered with racially marginalized communities to center their priorities, develop research to address health inequities, and disrupt traditional research models in health research institutions.[6,9,12] Over the past 3 decades, CBPR has evolved into a research approach that—when carried out according to its core principles—embraces antiracism principles and can be a tool to help dismantle structural racism in the United States. Even in this acknowledgment of CBPR's potential as an antiracist tool that can disrupt White supremacy, it was indeed the capital of White scholars that allowed this movement to gain acceptance and grow in academia. We hold these 2 truths to be in tension.

We argue that health research institutions should invest in research that funds and is led by racially marginalized communities, helps disrupt racial hierarchies, and contributes to transforming systems, structures, and institutions that are deeply implicated in reproducing racism. We cannot exhaustively cover all of the issues in this essay nor do we have all the answers; however, we hope to help our field move closer to transforming institutional practices that reproduce and reinforce racial inequities.

RESEARCH–ANTIRACIST PRINCIPLE SYNERGY

Synergies between a CBPR approach to research and antiracist approaches provide an opportunity for addressing racial inequities in institutions of higher education and traditional research practices. Camara Phyllis Jones, leading scholar of racism and health, has defined racism as

> a *system of structuring opportunity and assigning value based* on the social interpretation of how one looks, that unfairly disadvantages some individuals and communities, unfairly advantages other individuals and communities, and saps the strength of the whole society through *the waste of human resources*.[4(p231; emphasis added)]

Thus, health research that is antiracist would need to restructure opportunities, reassign value, and prevent the waste of human resources. The core principles of CBPR (Box 1) are intended to guide researchers to do exactly that.

CBPR principles aim to restructure opportunities by enhancing opportunities for community members and organizations to build solutions to community challenges, develop research questions, collaborate on data collection and analysis, and implement strategies for addressing inequities.[8,9,12] CBPR's explicit focus on capacity building by all team members provides opportunities for community members to build their research skill set, for academic researchers to learn community-centered skills

BOX 1— Principles for Community-Based Participatory Research

1. Recognizes community as a unit of identity
2. Builds on strengths and resources in the community
3. Facilitates a collaborative, equitable partnership in all phases of research, involving an empowering and power sharing process that attends to social inequalities
4. Fosters colearning and capacity building among all partners
5. Integrates and achieves a balance between knowledge generation and intervention for the mutual benefit of all partners
6. Focuses on the local relevance of public health problems and ecological perspectives that attend to the multiple determinants of health
7. Involves systems development using a cyclical and iterative process
8. Disseminates results to all partners and involves them in the wider dissemination of results
9. Involves a long-term process and commitment to sustainability
10. Openly addresses issues of race, ethnicity, racism, and social class and embodies "cultural humility"
11. Works to ensure research rigor and validity but also seeks to "broaden the bandwidth of validity" with respect to research relevance

Source. Israel et al.,[8] Minker and Wallerstein,[9] and Israel et al.[12]

and knowledge, and for all partners to examine the ways that institutionalized, personally mediated and internalized forms of racism affect collaborative work.[4,12] CBPR teams are also intentional about expanding space for community members to be experts on the project and topic. Beyond opportunities for individuals, CBPR creates opportunities for entire communities by budgeting financial resources to community-based organizations to strengthen capacity for community change. It also entails a critical evaluation of the balance of resources applied to research and those applied to action to create change based on research findings.

CBPR approaches work to reassign values by valuing and centering community perspectives more explicitly than they are in conventional research practices. CBPR principles emphasize that expertise lies in communities and places high value on the people and perspectives in racially marginalized communities. In practice, CBPR projects and partnerships are frequently the site of advocacy, policy change, and action related to injustices (e.g., environmental racism, incarceration, and policing) prioritized by racially marginalized communities.[13]

Finally, CBPR aims to prevent the waste of human resources by creating a research structure that explicitly challenges the marginalization of scholars and communities of color and the devaluation of their knowledge. Core CBPR practices aim to do this by channeling resources from well-financed predominantly White institutions into racially marginalized communities and by creating explicit opportunities to support community capacity for both research and action.

A CBPR approach also aligns with the leading antiracism framework for health research developed by Ford and Airhihenbuwa[21]: public health critical race praxis (PHCR). PHCR was developed to identify, understand, and undo the root causes of racial hierarchies and applies principles from critical race theory (CRT) to antiracist health research.

PHCR draws on fundamental pillars of CRT to emphasize the acknowledgment of the systemic White supremacy that operates at every level of US society.[21,22] PHCR also pulls from CRT in the recognition that we need to "center the margins" for an effective antiracist praxis. PHCR and CRT are also guided by Crenshaw's and other Black feminist scholars' concept of intersectionality, which was developed in recognition of the combined and often multiplicative impact of intersectional systems (e.g., economic structures, race, culture, and gender)[22] and was later applied to analysis of health outcomes.[23] PHCR and CRT emphasize questioning objectivity, questioning the evidence, and generating knowledge from perspectives that reside outside of the academy.

In Table 1, we show selected core principles and definitions from Ford and Airhihenbuwa's PHCR methodology.[21] For each PHCR principle (drawn from CRT concepts), we demonstrate alignments with guiding principles in CBPR. In Table A (available as a supplement to the online version of this article at http://www.ajph.org), we include all the core PHCR principles.

It is important to note that not all CBPR partnerships prioritize the study of racial influences on health outcomes (e.g., "primacy" from PHCR principles in Table 1). Rather, some partnerships focus on disrupting other systems of oppression, such as patriarchy, colonization, and heteronormativity, that often interlock with racism.[23] In addition, it is critical that CBPR partnerships discuss and determine the principles that will guide their work, including the integration of PHCR and CBPR principles relevant for their goals and context. As a result, principles will vary across partnerships.[8] Nonetheless, CBPR's focus on centering marginalized communities and disrupting various forms of inequities is consistent with PHCR principles.

CHALLENGES IN OUR CURRENT ENVIRONMENT

> "White supremacy is not a shark; it is the water."
>
> —*El Guante*

The waters of White supremacy in which we swim[24] pose major barriers to actualizing antiracist CBPR partnerships for health. These waters have been created and constructed over centuries to value the lives, institutions, and knowledge of White people and devalue the human dignity and lives of Black, Indigenous, Latinx, Arab, Asian, and other marginalized groups. In this sense, the impact of any programmatic or policy-based intervention is bound by linked oppressive systems.[15] The potential impact of CBPR on health equity is bound by larger oppressive systems' impact on resource and power distribution.

These waters are why both the NIH and US philanthropies dramatically underfund sickle cell disease—a disease predominantly afflicting Black Americans—compared with similar diseases that have a greater impact on Whites.[15,25] It is why the NIH has hardly invested in research on structural racism, despite it being a fundamental cause of so much death and disease.[5,26] It is why there is limited growth in public health faculty racial diversity, especially at research-intensive institutions and in tenured

TABLE 1— Selected List of Public Health Critical Race Methodology Principles and Application to CBPR Principles

PHCR Principle[a]	PHCR Principle Definition[a]	Application to CBPR Principles
Race consciousness	Deep awareness of one's racial position; awareness of racial stratification processes operating in a colorblind context	Focuses on equitable academic–community partnerships that recognize and attend to racial (and other) inequities; openly addresses racism (CBPR principles 3 and 10)
Primacy of racialization	Fundamental contribution of racial stratification to societal problems; central focus of CRT scholarship on explaining racial phenomena	Not all CBPR partnerships focus on racialization and racism; however, most work with communities of color and openly address issues of race, ethnicity, and racism (CBPR principle 10) often as these intersect with other dimensions of inequality (e.g., gender, class)
Ordinariness of racism	Racism is embedded in the social fabric of society	CBPR principles do not explicitly state this but aim to explicitly discuss issues of racism (CBPR principle 10); recognize and attend to power dynamics caused by racism in partnerships (CBPR principle 3)
Structural determinism	The fundamental role of macrolevel forces in driving and sustaining inequities across time and contexts	CBPR explicitly focuses on an ecological perspective that recognizes macrolevel forces as fundamental for causing inequities (CBPR principle 6) and attends to power dynamics rooted in racism that occur in partnerships (CBPR principle 3)
Social construction of knowledge	Established knowledge in a discipline can be reevaluated using antiracism modes of analysis	CBPR principles explicitly value and seek knowledge based in communities that may be different than traditional academic knowledge (CBPR principles 2, 4, and 5)
Intersectionality	Interlocking nature of cooccurring social categories (e.g., race, gender) and the forms of social stratification that maintain them	CBPR principles do not explicitly state this but aim to explicitly discuss issues of racism and social class (CBPR principle 10) and recognize and attend to power dynamics caused by social inequalities that occur in partnerships (CBPR principle 3)
Voice	Prioritizing the perspectives of marginalized persons; privileging the experiential knowledge of outsiders within	CBPR often occurs in racially marginalized communities where community members are equal partners in the research decision-making (CBPR principle 3) and focuses on issues identified and prioritized by members of the community (CBPR principle 6)

Note. CBPR = community-based participatory research; CRT = critical race theory; PHCR = public health critical race praxis.

[a]This column is quoted directly from Table 1 in Ford and Airhihenbuwa.[21]

positions.[27] And it is why the overwhelming majority of budgets and indirect costs for multimillion-dollar racial health inequities research goes to historically and predominantly White research universities with predominantly White faculty instead of to racially marginalized communities, community-based organizations, or historically Black colleges and universities. We highlight a few of the barriers to an antiracist health research agenda.

First, current academic structures incentivize short-term profit for universities and center knowledge production in individual academic faculty members rather than incentivizing long-term investments in communities and community expertise.[14] Academic researchers who would like to conduct antiracist CBPR research are often discouraged because it is too slow, underfunded, perceived as service, or not perceived as rigorous science.[28] Universities often prioritize federal grant funding—especially in decisions about faculty hiring, tenure, and promotion—and thus can sometimes disincentivize academic-based researchers from creating equitable partnerships that share grant dollars with communities.[17] Academic researchers, especially those who are scholars of color, are sometimes forced to exit partnerships because they could not find a job that supported their research or that earned tenure or because they felt the university environment was too toxic.[29] This dynamic is exacerbated by "health equity tourists"—primarily White scholars—who opportunistically seize on expanded health equity funding or publishing opportunities to advance their careers despite a lack of expertise.[30] The commitment to antiracist research and CBPR principles often rests on the individual researchers rather than institutional commitment.

Second, the NIH and other large health research–funding institutions prioritize research that focuses on proximate causes of diseases, biology, and individual health outcomes and have less emphasis on understanding and intervening in the sociopolitical roots of health and inequality. Of the \$41.7 billion in NIH funding in 2020, just 7% fit into the broad NIH-defined category of social determinants of health research.[31] (Most of the research categorized by the NIH as social determinants of health does not engage with the sociopolitical roots of health and does not adequately account for structural racism.[32]) CBPR partnerships aim to follow community priorities for research and intervention, but the pool of funding available severely constrains those choices. For example, in many cases, communities would prioritize ending police harassment and imprisonment of their residents,[26] but the funding agencies with the largest health research budgets continue to focus on proximal causes and medical solutions, rather than addressing the root causes of harm to racially marginalized communities.[31]

Third, there are substantial barriers—attributable to structural racism—that inhibit racially marginalized scholars, first-generation college-educated researchers, and community partners from receiving competitive research grants for large-scale funding.[5] Often (but certainly not always), academic researchers work for predominantly White institutions located outside the communities with whom they partner.[10] They are also often spawned from legacies of educational White privilege or do not belong to communities most affected by racial health inequities. Additionally, scholars from racially marginalized communities are often dissuaded from conducting research in partnership with their own community because it is unfairly perceived as biased.[29,33] Meanwhile, White academics are rewarded for conducting health research with these same communities.[30] Collectively, these inequitable practices systematically advantage White researchers and simultaneously discredit and marginalize scholars of color—a dual function of White supremacy in the academy.

Finally, CBPR partnerships occur in a White supremacy culture that places values on certain forms of knowledge prominent in predominantly White institutions and devalues those coming from institutions in racially marginalized communities. Excellent CBPR research is conducted by researchers at historically Black colleges and universities but does not receive the same recognition and support.[34] Despite the intentions of CBPR principles to center members of racially marginalized communities as experts with valuable knowledge, the society we live in—and our very own research institutions—continues to call on experts based in predominantly White universities to provide input on what is happening in racially marginalized communities.

These are but a few of the structural barriers CBPR partnerships face in living up to their principles. With these in mind, we recognize CBPR principles as aspirational, commonly eroded, or compromised because of the institutional and societal challenges described. They also represent a set of tools and perspectives that can help to chip away at the very structural barriers just described. Indeed, CBPR partnerships have played an important role in shifting institutions and policies, which we describe in several examples in the next section.

PARTNERSHIP AND ADVOCACY EXAMPLES

These examples—most of which are unpublished because of some of the barriers described in the preceding section—draw on the experiences of the authors.

Advocating in Local Government

A CBPR partnership in Flint, Michigan, played a fundamental role in the Genesee County, Michigan, government declaring racism a public health crisis on June 10, 2020, and the subsequent work to act based on the declaration. Researchers from Michigan State University and the University of Michigan–Flint worked in partnership with the Faith Subcommittee of the Greater Flint COVID-19 Taskforce on Racial Inequities and the community-based organization partners to conduct focus groups and community dialogues that informed a strategic plan for the county government to act on their declaration. This CBPR partnership had an antiracist outcome because it resulted in antiracist policy changes, such as a line item in the budget to support antiracism training, education, and initiatives.

Transformation in Universities

To build the cadre of underrepresented scholars of color in health research, the Transdisciplinary Research, Equity and Engagement (TREE) Center at the University of New Mexico is shifting the conditions for CBPR partnerships between scholars of color and communities of color. Scholars of color are supported by an academic and community of color mentor from the development of competitive pilot project proposals to the implementation of interventions in real-world settings as a model for centering community voice and building new lines of inquiry toward racial healing, social justice, and health equity. The TREE Center fosters the development of scholars of color by providing a community of mentors across 12 disciplines in the health and social sciences. A formal training and technical assistance program provides support for academic success (e.g., preparing tenure and promotion portfolios, development, and review of research proposals). The TREE Center also develops tools for engagement with communities that shift power dynamics and advocate changes in university procedures and policies that incentivize CBPR scholars.

Changing Funding Models

In the early 2000s, the National Center for Minority Health and Health Disparities convened a group of CBPR experts from across the United States to advise them in establishing a CBPR program at the center (subsequently "institute"). It incorporated a primary recommendation of the advisory group, which was the creation of a 3-phase funding cycle spanning an 11-year period. The 3 phases were (1) an initial 3-year planning and pilot project grant, (2) a 5-year intervention implementation grant, and (3) a 3-year dissemination grant to share findings and lessons learned. This extended timing allowed CBPR partnerships the time and resources needed to genuinely follow CBPR principles. This example of CBPR researchers advocating institutional transformation follows the PHCR and CRT concepts of "disciplinary self-critique" and "structural determinism" in that status quo norms at the NIH are perpetuating inequities in health research processes.

Another example of this is how at the urging of CBPR scholars and environmental justice advocates, the National Institute of Environmental Health Sciences (NIEHS) has experimented with innovations that shift power as part of their Research to Action program. The Environmental Justice: Partnerships for Communication program request for proposals sought to amplify community voices in identifying and defining problems related to environmental exposures, shaping research approaches to the problem, and setting priorities for intervention strategies. Particularly notable was that the study section that NIEHS convened for this funding mechanism included both academic-based researchers and environmental justice advocates to examine the science, the distribution of funds, and whether proposals reflected community priorities. This example follows principles from PHCR and CRT because it shifted the voices of environmental justice advocates from the margins to the center to shift funding processes and outcomes.

Finally, Tribal nations and Native scholars across the United States have recently challenged White supremacy by demanding cultural-centered CBPR and Indigenous-led research through 2 NIH initiatives: the Native American Research Centers for Health and the Intervention Research to Improve Native American Health (IRINAH) funding. A major goal has been to center funding in Native communities and organizations and increase the number of Native scholars and their success in the academy, including increased access to R01 (research project grant) funding. For more about the IRINAH initiative, see the special issue in *Prevention Science*.[7] Although Native scholars have begun to replace their White colleagues as principal investigators, the NIH has not yet adopted a similar initiative for other scholars of color. Like the previous examples, this example of CBPR research draws on PHCR and CRT principles of centering the margins and disciplinary self-critique to create antiracist processes for conducting research.

RECOMMENDATIONS AND CONSIDERATIONS

In the short term, research funders should shift substantial funds to focusing on structural racism and encouraging research approaches that align with both antiracism and CBPR principles. A recent request for applications from the NIH for projects with the goal of "understanding and addressing the impact of structural racism" focused funding on racism but did not take an explicitly antiracist approach to how funding decisions were made or which types of projects were eligible for funding. These types of funding opportunities are limited and are subject to the whims of new federal leadership because they are not institutionalized. Most universities and research institutions are motivated by funding, and thus if funders transform how they allocate resources they can also transform these academic research institutions.

The examples we have provided show how CBPR researchers can advocate funding mechanisms to facilitate long-term commitments with racially marginalized communities. In addition, ensuring that NIH and other funders' funding decisions are shaped by members of racially marginalized communities—like the NIEHS study section example—can help make sure that funding provides community resources and focuses on fundamental causes of multiple health issues (e.g., systems of incarceration, finance, policing, environmental protection, housing).

Longer term, we need to work toward a future in which racially marginalized communities are allocating and receiving public funding and directing antiracist health research that can have an impact on their own communities.[35] This change will require fundamental transformation in how universities operate and how research is defined, originated, and funded. Substantial rethinking and reorientation among research institutions to shift funding allocations will be required to ensure that funds are available to support action to address the inequities that are the focus of the research. The research to action mechanism described in the preceding section is an example of such a funding mechanism. There is a critical need for focused attention to expand and create additional mechanisms for directing funding to support antiracist actions.

Accountability to Communities of Color

Long-term commitment and community-driven policy change can enhance trust and accountability with communities of color, an essential aspect of antiracist praxis. Universities and other research institutions that are committed to antiracist practices need to build in measures of accountability to communities affected by racism and racial health inequities. Long-term commitment is a key principle of CBPR partnerships, and we need institutional support for larger partnerships between universities and communities and cities to help ensure the long-term sustainability of CBPR research. Such partnerships might be established in the form of community–academic centers or institutes (e.g., the TREE Center or the Detroit Urban Research Center), which extend beyond any single externally funded project. Ideally these would have university funding for core infrastructure support in addition to external funding to foster, promote, and build capacity to conduct antiracist CBPR.

It is essential to build in accountability metrics and mechanisms to ensure a continued focus on social impact to address structural racism. A practical model for social change links research efforts to policy change to transform the racial structures through distributive, procedural, and restorative justice approaches that remediate unfair policies.[13,36,37] Examples include working to ensure that indirect costs received as part of grant funding are equitably invested in communities instead of adding solely to a university's budget, dedicating a portion of project funds to scholarships for community youths, and demanding that universities divest from companies and other institutions that harm their community through, for example, incarceration or climate change. These forms of accountability can help move research institutions into closer alignment with antiracist and CBPR principles and ultimately help disrupt structural racism and White supremacy. These types of actions—and not just platitudes—can help to build trust over time.

Reflection and Adaptation

Given that racism adapts over time, antiracist CBPR approaches will also need to adapt over time. CBPR principles of colearning and capacity building—and openly addressing issues of racism and social classism—require CBPR researchers and community partners to follow guided approaches that allow continued critical self-reflection and collective reflection regarding racial equity in the partnership.[10] Being adaptive means that the current CBPR core principles may and should be revised in the future to better align with community priorities or antiracism ideas. Dialogues will be essential in partnerships, recognizing that racism is shaped by local histories and relationships, and thus will vary not only over time but by location.[38,39]

In this reflection, we cannot overlook that the development of CBPR approaches has historically been led in academia predominantly by White scholars. Many of the authors of this essay benefit from the waters of White supremacy while simultaneously fighting for the CBPR partnerships and principles that swim against the currents. Given the racism embedded in the academy, White scholars' ideas have been more likely to be legitimized and shared. Furthermore, in some instances the voices of scholars of color are marginalized when they are relinquished to secondary authors or investigators in funded research with communities of color.[29,33] The future of antiracist CBPR needs to own and address this dynamic. Candid reflection and courageous conversations regarding internalized privilege among White scholars and internalized oppression among scholars of color can facilitate processes of healing for racial justice in CBPR.

The possibilities for CBPR have been changing as Indigenous researchers and other scholars of color have advanced to senior positions in predominantly White institutions, as historically Black colleges and universities have made innovations in CBPR principles,[40] and as tribes and communities have demanded equitable distribution of resources and community-prioritized and -led decisions.[7] This is an opportunity to raise the critical nature of antiracism conversations in partnerships and demand change in academia and funding institutions.

CONCLUSIONS

Health research urgently needs to follow antiracist research principles.

Alignments between a CBPR approach and antiracist approaches provide a path toward addressing historical and contemporary racial inequities embedded in institutions of higher education and in traditional research processes. Achieving racial justice and ameliorating inequities is a call to action for the field of health research to address racism in health research, center scholars and communities of color, and work together as intercultural allies in confronting White supremacy with focused deliberative action toward racial healing, justice, and reconciliation. AJPH

ABOUT THE AUTHORS

Paul J. Fleming, Melissa S. Creary, Barbara A. Israel, and Amy J. Schulz are with the School of Public Health, University of Michigan, Ann Arbor. Lisa Cacari Stone and Nina Wallerstein are with the College of Population Health, University of New Mexico, Albuquerque. Ella Greene-Moton is with Community Based Organizations Partners, Flint, MI. Kent D. Key is with the Division of Public Health, Michigan State University, East Lansing. Angela G. Reyes is with the Detroit Hispanic Development Corporation, Detroit, MI.

CORRESPONDENCE

Correspondence should be sent to Paul J. Fleming, 1415 Washington Heights, Ann Arbor, MI 48109-2029 (e-mail: pauljf@umich.edu). Reprints can be ordered at http://www.ajph.org by clicking the "Reprints" link.

PUBLICATION INFORMATION

Full Citation: Fleming PJ, Cacari Stone L, Creary MS, et al. Antiracism and community-based participatory research: synergies, challenges, and opportunities. *Am J Public Health*. 2023;113(1):70–78.

Acceptance Date: August 30, 2022.

DOI: https://doi.org/10.2105/AJPH.2022.307114

CONTRIBUTORS

P. J. Fleming led the writing and revisions of the article. P. J. Fleming, L. Cacari Stone, and A. J. Schulz drafted substantial portions of the text. All authors conceptualized the article, contributed ideas, and critically edited and revised the article.

ACKNOWLEDGMENTS

This work was supported by the National Institute of Minority Health and Health Disparities (grant U54 MD004811-08) for support of the Transdisciplinary Research, Equity and Engagement Center; the National Institute for Environmental Health Research (grants R01ES032389, P30 ES017885); the National Institute of Nursing Research (grant R01NR016123); the National Institute of Minority Health and Health Disparities (grant K01MD015079); and the National Center for Institutional Diversity, University of Michigan.

Note. The content of this editorial is solely the responsibility of the authors and does not necessarily represent the official views of the funders.

CONFLICTS OF INTEREST

The authors have no conflicts of interest to declare.

HUMAN PARTICIPANT PROTECTION

No protocol approval was necessary because no human participants were involved in this article.

REFERENCES

1. Minkler M, Blackwell AG, Thompson M, Tamir H. Community-based participatory research: implications for public health funding. *Am J Public Health*. 2003;93(8):1210–1213. https://doi.org/10.2105/AJPH.93.8.1210
2. Yonas MA, Jones N, Eng E, et al. The art and science of integrating Undoing Racism with CBPR: challenges of pursuing the NIH funding to investigate cancer care and racial equity. *J Urban Health*. 2006;83(6):1004–1012. https://doi.org/10.1007/s11524-006-9114-x
3. National Institutes of Health. UNITE. February 24, 2021. Available at: https://www.nih.gov/ending-structural-racism/unite. Accessed September 30, 2021.
4. Jones CP. Toward the science and practice of anti-racism: launching a national campaign against racism. *Ethn Dis*. 2018;28(suppl 1):231–234. https://doi.org/10.18865/ed.28.S1.231
5. Kaiser J. NIH apologizes for "structural racism," pledges change. *Science*. 2021;371(6533):977. https://doi.org/10.1126/science.371.6533.977
6. Nguyen TT, Wallerstein N, Das R, et al. Conducting community-based participatory research with minority communities to reduce health disparities. In: Dankwa-Mullan I, Perez-Stable EJ, Gardner KL, Zhang X, Rosario AM, eds. *The Science of Health Disparities Research*. Hoboken, NJ: Wiley; 2021:171–186. https://doi.org/10.1002/9781119374855.ch11
7. Crump AD, Etz K, Arroyo JA, Hemberger N, Srinivasan S. Accelerating and strengthening Native American health research through a collaborative NIH Initiative. *Prev Sci*. 2020;21(1):1–4. https://doi.org/10.1007/s11121-017-0854-5
8. Israel BA, Schulz AJ, Coombe C, et al. Community-based participatory research: an approach to research in the urban context. In: Galea S, Ettman C, & Vlahov D, eds. *Urban Health*. Oxford, UK: Oxford University Press; 2019:272–282.
9. Minkler M, Wallerstein NB, eds. *Community-Based Participatory Research for Health: From Process to Outcomes*, 2nd edition. San Francisco, CA: Jossey-Bass; 2008.
10. Muhammad M, Wallerstein N, Sussman AL, Avila M, Belone L, Duran B. Reflections on researcher identity and power: the impact of positionality on community based participatory research (CBPR) processes and outcomes. *Crit Sociol*. 2015; 41(7–8):1045–1063. https://doi.org/10.1177/0896920513516025
11. Salimi Y, Shahandeh K, Malekafzali H, et al. Is community-based participatory research (CBPR) useful? A systematic review on papers in a decade. *Int J Prev Med*. 2012;3(6):386–393.
12. Israel BA, Schulz AJ, Parker EA, Becker AB. Review of community-based research: assessing partnership approaches to improve public health. *Annu Rev Public Health*. 1998;19:173–202. https://doi.org/10.1146/annurev.publhealth.19.1.173
13. Minkler M. Linking science and policy through community-based participatory research to study and address health disparities. *Am J Public Health*. 2010;100(suppl 1):S81–S87. https://doi.org/10.2105/AJPH.2009.165720
14. Flicker S, Travers R, Guta A, McDonald S, Meagher A. Ethical dilemmas in community-based participatory research: recommendations for institutional review boards. *J Urban Health*. 2007;84(4):478–493. https://doi.org/10.1007/s11524-007-9165-7
15. Creary MS. Bounded justice and the limits of health equity. *J Law Med Ethics*. 2021;49(2): 241–256. https://doi.org/10.1017/jme.2021.34
16. Bailey ZD, Krieger N, Agénor M, Graves J, Linos N, Bassett MT. Structural racism and health inequities in the USA: evidence and interventions. *Lancet*. 2017;389(10077):1453–1463. https://doi.org/10.1016/S0140-6736(17)30569-X
17. Woolford SJ, Buyuktur AG, Piechowski P, Doshi A, Marsh EE. Critical barriers to effective community–academic research partnerships and potential solutions. *J Clin Transl Sci*. 2019; 3(suppl 1):86–87. https://doi.org/10.1017/cts.2019.199
18. Wallerstein N, Duran B. Theoretical, historical and practice roots of CBPR. In: Wallerstein N, Duran B, Oetzel JG, Minkler M, eds. *Community-Based Participatory Research for Health: Advancing Social and Health Equity*. San Francisco, CA: Jossey-Bass; 2017:17–29.
19. Freire P. Creating alternative research methods: learning to do it by doing it. In: Hall B, Gillette A, Tandon R, eds. *Creating Knowledge: A Monopoly? Participatory Research in Development*. New Delhi, India: Society for Participatory Research in Asia; 1982:29–40.
20. Sousa Santos, B de. *Epistemologies of the South: Justice Against Epistemicide*. New York, NY: Routledge; 2015. https://doi.org/10.4324/9781315634876
21. Ford CL, Airhihenbuwa CO. The public health critical race methodology: praxis for antiracism research. *Social Science & Medicine*. 2010;71(8): 1390–1398. https://doi.org/10.1016/j.socscimed.2010.07.030
22. Crenshaw K, Gotanda N, Peller G, Thomas K, eds. *Critical Race Theory: The Key Writings That Formed the Movement*. New York, NY: New Press; 1995.
23. Mullings L, Schulz AJ. *Gender, Race, Class, and Health: Intersectional Approaches*. San Francisco, CA: Jossey-Bass; 2006.
24. Alang S, Hardeman R, Karbeah J, et al. White supremacy and the core functions of public health. *Am J Public Health*. 2021;111(5):815–819. https://doi.org/10.2105/AJPH.2020.306137

25. Farooq F, Mogayzel PJ, Lanzkron S, Haywood C, Strouse JJ. Comparison of US federal and foundation funding of research for sickle cell disease and cystic fibrosis and factors associated with research productivity. *JAMA Netw Open.* 2020; 3(3):e201737. https://doi.org/10.1001/jamanetworkopen.2020.1737
26. Fleming PJ, Spolum MM, Lopez WD, Galea S. The public health funding paradox: how funding the problem and solution impedes public health progress. *Public Health Rep.* 2021;136(1):10–13. https://doi.org/10.1177/0033354920969172
27. Goodman MS, Plepys CM, Bather JR, Kelliher RM, Healton CG. Racial/Ethnic diversity in academic public health: 20-year update. *Public Health Rep.* 2020;135(1):74–81. https://doi.org/10.1177/0033354919887747
28. Lowry KW, Ford-Paz R. Early career academic researchers and community-based participatory research: wrestling match or dancing partners? *Clin Transl Sci.* 2013;6(6):490–492. https://doi.org/10.1111/cts.12045
29. Subbaraman N. How #BlackInTheIvory put a spotlight on racism in academia. *Nature.* 2020; 582(7812):327–328. https://doi.org/10.1038/d41586-020-01741-7
30. Lett E, Adekunle D, McMurray P, et al. Health equity tourism: ravaging the justice landscape. *J Med Syst.* 2022;46(3):17. https://doi.org/10.1007/s10916-022-01803-5
31. National Institutes of Health. Estimates of funding for various research, condition, and disease categories (RCDC). Available at: https://report.nih.gov/funding/categorical-spending#. Accessed September 30, 2021.
32. Yearby R. Structural racism and health disparities: reconfiguring the social determinants of health framework to include the root cause. *J Law Med Ethics.* 2020;48(3):518–526. https://doi.org/10.1177/1073110520958876
33. Frazier KN. Academic bullying: a barrier to tenure and promotion for African-American faculty. *Florida Journal of Educational Administration & Policy.* 2011;5(1):1–13.
34. Sydnor KD, Hawkins AS, Edwards LV. Expanding research opportunities: making the argument for the fit between HBCUs and community-based participatory research. *J Negro Educ.* 2010;79(1): 79–86.
35. Stoecker R. Are academics irrelevant? Roles for scholars in participatory research. *Am Behav Sci.* 1999;42(5):840–854. https://doi.org/10.1177/00027649921954561
36. Coombe CM, Schulz AJ, Guluma L, et al. Enhancing capacity of community–academic partnerships to achieve health equity: results from the CBPR partnership academy. *Health Promot Pract.* 2020;21(4):552–563. https://doi.org/10.1177/1524839918818830
37. Cacari Stone L, Pastor M, Griffin J, Minkler M. Moving the policy dial through equity-focused community organizing. In: Minkler M, Wakimoto P, eds. *Community Organizing and Community Building for Health and Welfare.* New Brunswick, NJ: Rutgers University Press; 2012:385–400.
38. Cacari-Stone L, Wallerstein N, Garcia AP, Minkler M. The promise of community-based participatory research for health equity: a conceptual model for bridging evidence with policy. *Am J Public Health.* 2014;104(9):1615–1623. https://doi.org/10.2105/AJPH.2014.301961
39. Muhammad M, Garzón C, Reyes A, The West Oakland Environmental Indicators Project. Understanding contemporary racism, power, and privilege and their impacts on CBPR. In: Wallerstein N, Duran B, Oetzel J, Minkler M, eds. *Community-Based Participatory Research for Health: Advancing Social and Health Equity.* San Francisco, CA: Jossey-Bass; 2018:47–59.
40. Braithwaite RL, Akintobi TH, Blumenthal DS, Langley WM. *The Morehouse Model: How One School of Medicine Revolutionized Community Engagement and Health Equity.* Baltimore, MD: Johns Hopkins University Press; 2020.

Timing and Trends for Municipal Wastewater, Lab-Confirmed Case, and Syndromic Case Surveillance of COVID-19 in Raleigh, North Carolina

Nadine Kotlarz, PhD, David A. Holcomb, PhD, A. B. M. Tanvir Pasha, MS, Stacie Reckling, EA, Judith Kays, Yi-Chun Lai, PhD, Sean Daly, Sivaranjani Palani, Erika Bailey, Virginia T. Guidry, PhD, Ariel Christensen, Steven Berkowitz, Jane A. Hoppin, ScD, Helena Mitasova, PhD, Lawrence S. Engel, PhD, Francis L. de los Reyes III, PhD, and Angela Harris, PhD

See also Keck and Berry, p. 6.

Objectives. To compare 4 COVID-19 surveillance metrics in a major metropolitan area.

Methods. We analyzed severe acute respiratory syndrome coronavirus 2 (SARS-CoV-2) RNA in wastewater influent and primary solids in Raleigh, North Carolina, from April 10 through December 13, 2020. We compared wastewater results with lab-confirmed COVID-19 cases and syndromic COVID-like illness (CLI) cases to answer 3 questions: (1) Did they correlate? (2) What was the temporal alignment of the different surveillance systems? (3) Did periods of significant change (i.e., trends) align?

Results. In the Raleigh sewershed, wastewater influent, wastewater primary solids, lab-confirmed cases, and CLI were strongly or moderately correlated. Trends in lab-confirmed cases and wastewater influent were observed earlier, followed by CLI and, lastly, wastewater primary solids. All 4 metrics showed sustained increases in COVID-19 in June, July, and November 2020 and sustained decreases in August and September 2020.

Conclusions. In a major metropolitan area in 2020, the timing of and trends in municipal wastewater, lab-confirmed case, and syndromic case surveillance of COVID-19 were in general agreement.

Public Health Implications. Our results provide evidence for investment in SARS-CoV-2 wastewater and CLI surveillance to complement information provided through lab-confirmed cases. (*Am J Public Health*. 2023;113(1):79–88. https://doi.org/10.2105/AJPH.2022.307108)

AJPH January 2023, Vol 113, No. 1

COVID-19 public health surveillance relies on multiple data sources to estimate disease burden. The number of positive clinical tests over time has served as a primary metric for tracking COVID-19 infections in North Carolina because clinical testing of individuals accurately identifies cases and is legally required for surveillance of reportable diseases, including COVID-19.[1] Clinical testing is, however, costly and inefficient as a means of population-level surveillance of COVID-19.[2] In addition, this metric can be limited by sensitivity,[3] clinical test availability,[4] and changes in testing behavior such as the rise in use of nonreportable, at-home rapid test kits.[5]

Surveillance of severe acute respiratory syndrome coronavirus 2 (SARS-CoV-2) RNA in wastewater influent or settled wastewater solids has gained traction in public health practice.[6] In addition to capturing data on symptomatic individuals who are likely to be tested, wastewater surveillance captures information on infections among asymptomatic carriers who shed the virus in feces but are less likely to be tested (Figure 1). In retrospective studies, SARS-CoV-2 RNA concentrations in wastewater have been shown to correlate positively with reported clinical COVID-19 cases.[7,8] Public health officials have used wastewater surveillance trends to target public health mitigation efforts.[9] Most wastewater surveillance is conducted using centralized wastewater treatment systems; wastewater surveillance is not as efficient in communities

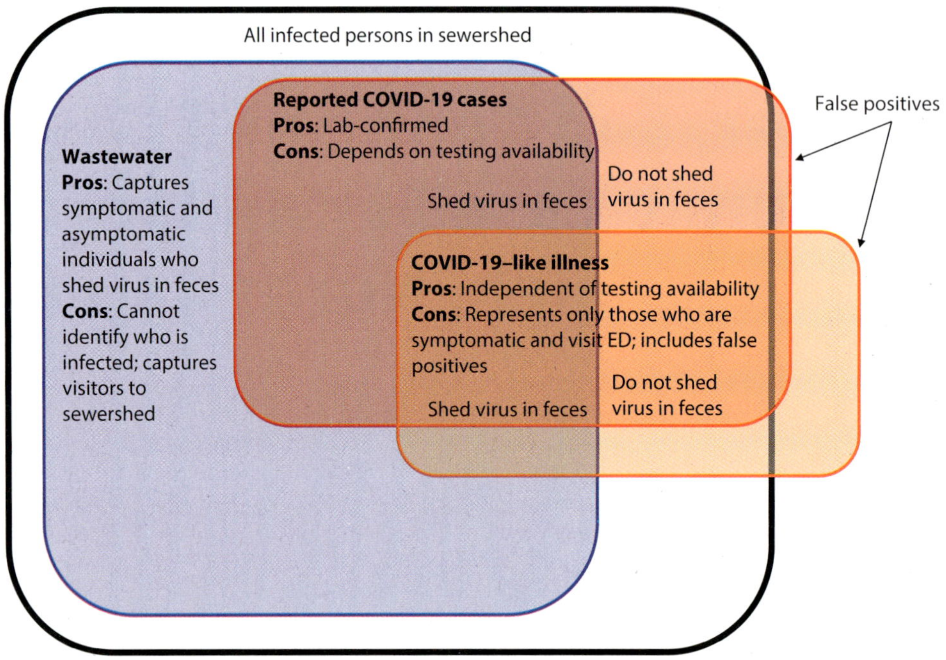

FIGURE 1— Depiction of Populations Captured by COVID-19 Surveillance Systems

Note. ED = emergency department; SARS-CoV-2 = severe acute respiratory syndrome coronavirus 2. The black box contains all SARS-CoV-2 infections in the sewershed. Infected individuals who shed the virus in feces contribute to SARS-CoV-2 RNA levels in wastewater (blue). Data on individuals seeking diagnostic testing are captured through reportable communicable disease surveillance (red). Data on individuals exhibiting COVID-like illness (CLI) at an ED are captured through ED syndromic surveillance (orange). False positives are shown outside the black box (orange for CLI and red for diagnostic testing). All reported cases are estimates of true cases. Individuals who do not seek testing, visit an ED, or shed the virus in feces are not captured by these surveillance systems (i.e., the white space inside the black box).

with a high proportion of people dependent on individual septic systems.

Another form of surveillance used for COVID-19 response is syndromic surveillance for COVID-like illness (CLI) based on prediagnostic emergency department (ED) data not confirmed through laboratory testing. CLI captures data on individuals with serious illness and those seeking care at EDs, representing a smaller segment of the infected population. Syndromic surveillance is mandated in North Carolina[10] and is routinely used for other respiratory conditions, including influenza.

Given the different segments of the population captured via wastewater, lab-confirmed case, and CLI surveillance (Figure 1), it is important to evaluate how these surveillance systems compare in a given population. Wastewater may provide more sensitive surveillance of changing infection rates in areas where there is incomplete ascertainment of cases through clinical testing.[11] Increases in wastewater concentrations have sometimes preceded increases in clinical cases.[12] CLI surveillance based on ED data is unlikely to be more timely than lab-confirmed case surveillance, but it may be nearly as timely. With electronic health information systems, data on CLI ascertained at EDs can be available in near real time,[13] whereas laboratory testing can entail delays from sample collection to results reporting.

We compared COVID-19 surveillance data sets from a major metropolitan area and included 2 wastewater metrics. We analyzed SARS-CoV-2 RNA concentrations in wastewater influent and primary solids from a municipal wastewater treatment plant in Raleigh, NC. Subsequently, we compared wastewater levels with lab-confirmed COVID-19 and CLI counts for the sewershed to answer 3 questions: (1) Did they correlate? (2) What was the temporal alignment of the different surveillance systems? (3) Did trends (i.e., periods of significant increases or decreases) align across surveillance systems? This research can inform how public health officials look across surveillance systems to estimate COVID-19 burdens.

METHODS

Raw wastewater influent and primary clarifier solids (i.e., primary solids) were sampled from the Neuse River Resource Recovery Facility in Raleigh between April 10 and December 13, 2020. We collected 24-hour composite influent wastewater samples (100 or 500 mL) and grab samples of solids (40 mL) 2 or

3 times weekly, with some periods of daily sampling (102 dates in total; Figure A, available as a supplement to the online version of this article at https://ajph.org). This facility serves approximately 580 000 people and had average treated flows of 48 million gallons per day in 2020. Solids collected from primary clarifiers were predominantly influent solids, but waste-activated solids were also present because the facility co-settles waste-activated solids in its primary clarifiers. Although co-settling waste-activated solids in primary clarifiers is not a common wastewater treatment practice, it is a recognized practice for improved sludge thickening.[14,15] The residence time of solids in the clarifiers was, on average, 2.8 days (range = 1.8–4.3 days), which is longer than typical primary clarifier residence times (on the order of hours).

Concentrations of SARS-CoV-2 N1 and N2 genes in wastewater samples were determined via reverse-transcription-droplet digital polymerase chain reaction (see Supporting Information, available as a supplement to the online version of this article at https://ajph.org). Wastewater sample processing protocols, depicted in Figure B (influent; available as a supplement to the online version of this article at https://ajph.org) and Figure C (primary solids; available as a supplement to the online version of this article at https://ajph.org), incorporated several of the current best practices.[16] Normalized N1 results (Supporting Information) were used in subsequent analyses with lab-confirmed cases and CLI.

Lab-Confirmed COVID-19 Case Data

Individual-level lab-confirmed COVID-19 cases with residential addresses from the North Carolina Electronic Disease Surveillance System were provided by the North Carolina Department of Health and Human Services. Positive case counts included polymerase chain reaction–positive tests, antigen-positive tests, and a few polymerase chain reaction–negative tests determined to be positive cases based on physician case notes. Cleaned residential addresses were geocoded in ArcGIS Pro version 2.7.0 (ESRI, Redlands, CA) via the 2018 ESRI Business Analyst USA_LocalComposite locator (Supporting Information). As a means of producing daily case counts, we summed cases in the sewershed using specimen collection dates or test result report dates.

COVID-Like Illness Data

Data on individual-level CLI cases geocoded at the residential zip code level were acquired from the North Carolina Disease Event Tracking and Epidemiologic Collection Tool, a public health syndromic surveillance system capturing all civilian ED visits in North Carolina (as reporting is mandatory).[13] CLI ascertained at urgent care centers was not included because NC does not share these data with external researchers.

CLI was defined according to *International Statistical Classification of Diseases and Related Health Problems, 10th Revision* (*ICD-10*; Geneva, Switzerland: World Health Organization; 1992) diagnostic codes (B97.2 or B34.2, J12.81 or J12.82, or U07.1 or U07.2[17]) or 1 of the following conditions: a chief complaint related to coronavirus, triage notes indicating a loss of sense of taste or smell, or triage notes indicating shortness of breath with fever. CLI cases that also had diagnostic codes for influenza (J09–J11.89) were excluded unless they had 1 of the *ICD-10* inclusion codes. The date for each CLI record was the ED visit date. We estimated daily CLI counts in the sewershed by summing counts in each of the 27 zip codes located entirely or partially in the sewershed, weighted by population density according to 2010 census block data.

Correlation Analysis

We used Spearman's rank correlation to determine the relationship between wastewater SARS-CoV-2 N1 concentrations (in influent or primary solids) and lab-confirmed COVID-19 cases or CLI. To investigate temporal alignment, we compared correlation coefficients and identified the maximum coefficient as 1 data set was offset forward or backward in time relative to another data set.[18–22] To reduce variation in the measurements for this analysis, we used the rolling 3-sampling-event averages of normalized SARS-CoV-2 quantities in wastewater influent and primary solids and the rolling 7-day averages for lab-confirmed cases and CLI. We used 2000 resamples with replacement to calculate bootstrap 95% confidence intervals for the correlation coefficient at each lead or lag and for all pairwise differences between correlations.[23] Correlation pairs were considered significantly different if the Bonferroni-adjusted 95% confidence interval for their difference excluded 0.[24]

Distributed Lag Model

The distributed lag measurement error time series model is an accepted epidemiological model for time series data.[25] We adapted a Bayesian distributed lag model developed previously[8] as a secondary approach to investigate temporal alignment between SARS-CoV-2 RNA levels in wastewater influent or primary solids and changes in clinical case rates.

The 3-day rolling average of clinical cases was predicted via wastewater measurements from 3 sampling events before the report date until 3 sampling events after. A random effect was included in the model to account for overdispersion.

Trends

Trends were classified as increasing, decreasing, or plateau through a linear regression with observations from each surveillance system as the dependent variable and date as the independent variable; trend classification was based on slope (positive, negative, or 0) and statistical significance ($P<.05$).[6] We classified short-term and sustained trends using regressions of 3 data points (approximately 1 week in duration) and 7 data points (approximately 2 weeks), respectively.[26]

RESULTS

SARS-CoV-2 RNA was frequently detected in wastewater influent and solids during the 247-day study period (April 10 to Dec 13, 2020); influent samples had detectable levels of the SARS-CoV-2 N1 gene on 96 of 102 wastewater sampling dates (94%); solids samples had detectable N1 on all 102 days (Figure B). The SARS-CoV-2 N2 gene was detectable in influent on 94 of 102 days (92%) and solids on 100 of 102 days (98%). Because N1 and N2 gene concentrations were highly correlated in influent (Spearman $\rho=0.83$; $P<.001$) and solids ($\rho=0.93$, $P<.001$) and N1 had a slightly higher detection rate, we focused our subsequent analyses on N1.

Surveillance Data Set Correlations

SARS-CoV-2 RNA daily loads in influent and SARS-CoV-2 RNA concentrations in primary solids (Figure 2) were moderately correlated over the study period ($\rho=0.65$; $P<.001$; C). Wastewater influent was strongly correlated with lab-confirmed cases ($\rho=0.74$; $P<.001$; Figure 2; Figure D, available as a supplement to the online version of this article at https://ajph.org), as were wastewater primary solids ($\rho=0.71$; $P<.001$; Figure E and Table A, available as supplements to the online version of this article at https://ajph.org). Furthermore, wastewater influent was moderately correlated with CLI ($\rho=0.61$; $P<.001$; Figure 2; Figure F, available as a supplement to the online version of this article at https://ajph.org), whereas solids were strongly correlated with CLI ($\rho=0.71$; $P<.001$; Figure G, available as a supplement to the online version of this article at https://ajph.org).

The strongest correlation observed was between lab-confirmed cases and CLI ($\rho=0.84$; $P<.001$; Figure H, available as a supplement to the online version of this article at https://ajph.org); during the study period, there were 20 858 lab-confirmed COVID-19 cases and 7441 cases of CLI in the sewershed. Lab-confirmed cases and CLI were highly correlated in earlier and later portions of the study period (Table B, available as a supplement to the online version of this article at https://ajph.org). The earlier portion (April 10 through August 13, 2020) captured the first rise and fall of infections and was characterized by lower testing penetration[4] and fewer ED visits (Figure I, available as a supplement to the online version of this article at https://ajph.org). The correlations between cases of CLI and wastewater (influent and primary solids) were substantially higher earlier in the study period (Table B).

Temporal Comparisons

The strongest correlation between SARS-CoV-2 N1 daily load in wastewater influent and N1 concentrations in wastewater primary solids was found for solids samples collected 2 sampling events after influent (given our sampling frequency, 2 sampling events represented 5.9 ±1.2 days; $\rho=0.65$; Figure J, available as a supplement to the online version of this article at https://ajph.org).

Correlations between lab-confirmed cases and wastewater influent daily load increased slightly as cases were offset from 0 to 3 days ahead of the influent sample collection date, with the strongest correlation observed for case specimens collected 3 days before an influent sample ($\rho=0.75$; Figure 3). The median duration between specimen collection date and results report date was 1 day (5th–95th percentiles: 0–4 days). When report date for case results was used instead of specimen collection date, the strongest correlation between cases and wastewater influent was observed for cases reported on the same day that influent was sampled (i.e., day 0; $\rho=0.75$). For wastewater primary solids, correlations between solids concentrations and lab-confirmed cases increased gradually as cases were offset 0 days to 7 days ahead of solids, with the strongest correlation found for case specimens collected 7 days before a solids sample ($\rho=0.80$). This correlation was significantly higher than correlations for case specimens collected 1 to 7 days after a solids sample.

The strongest correlation between CLI and wastewater influent was found for CLI reported 3 days after an influent sample was collected ($\rho=0.64$; Figure 3). The strongest correlation between lab-confirmed cases and CLI was found for clinical case specimens collected 1 day before the ED visit date ($\rho=0.84$). This correlation was significantly higher

AJPH January 2023, Vol 113, No. 1

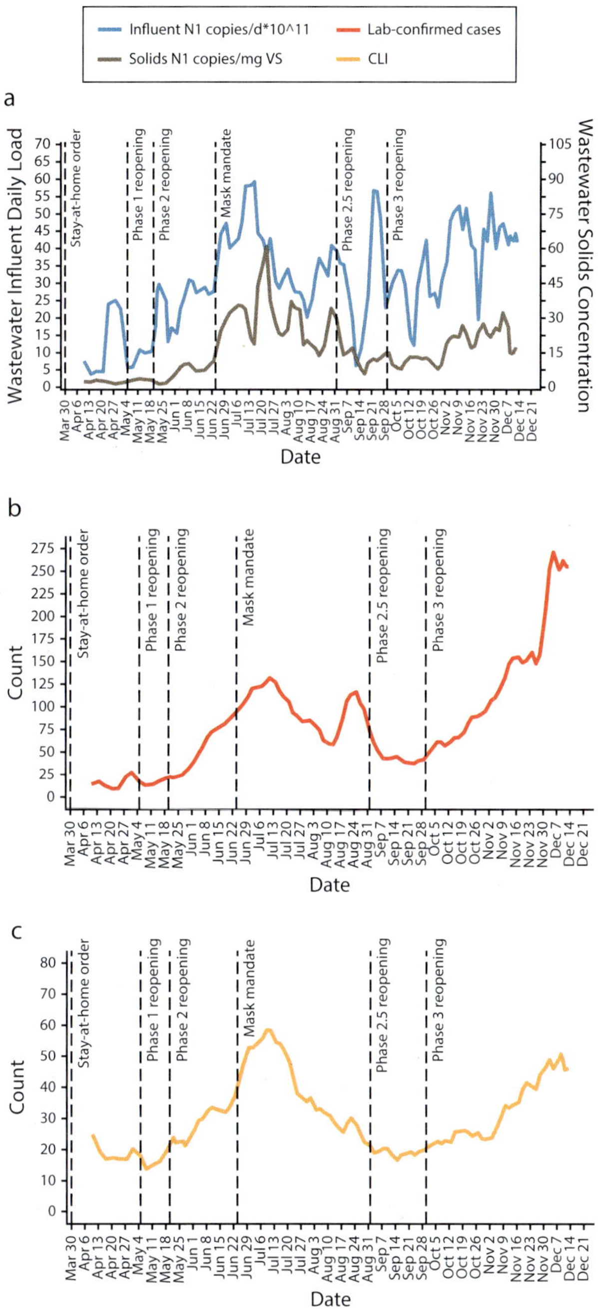

FIGURE 2— COVID-19 Surveillance Time Series for (a) Wastewater Influent and Primary Solids, (b) Lab-Confirmed Cases, and (c) CLI Cases: Raleigh, NC, Sewershed, April 10–December 13, 2020

Note. CLI = COVID-like illness. The wastewater influent and primary solids in panel a are 3-sampling-event averages (mean ±SD duration = 5.7 ±1.2 days). Lab-confirmed (panel b) and CLI (panel c) cases are 7-day averages of daily counts. Dotted lines indicate dates of North Carolina executive orders. The specimen collection date was used for cases and the date of emergency department visit for CLI.

than correlations for case specimens collected on the same day or up to 7 days after the ED visit date. Correlations were generally similar but slightly weaker for the surrounding days. Distributed lag modeling results were consistent with the correlation analysis with date offsets: wastewater influent and primary solids lagged clinical cases based on case specimen collection date (Table C, available as a supplement to the online version of this article at https://ajph.org).

Numbers of Significant Trends

Public health officials monitor for significant changes in levels of COVID-19 surveillance metrics to inform public health action.[27] Short-term or weekly trend monitoring is valuable because a short-term trend can be an early indicator of a sustained trend and because, particularly at the start of the pandemic, public health officials acted as quickly as possible. Across the different surveillance data sets, we might expect the numbers of trends to be similar but the temporal alignment to be shifted. However, lab-confirmed cases exhibited substantially more short-term increases (n = 17) than CLI (n = 10), wastewater primary solids (n = 7), and wastewater influent (n = 4) over the study period. Lab-confirmed cases had a number of periods of sustained increases (n = 51) similar to that of CLI (n = 45; within 20% of each other), but wastewater primary solids (n = 21) and wastewater influent had substantially fewer (n = 20).

In terms of periods of decreasing levels of COVID-19 metrics, the numbers of short-term decreases were greatest for lab-confirmed cases (n = 8) and wastewater solids (n = 7), followed by CLI (n = 5) and wastewater influent (n = 1). Furthermore, the numbers of sustained decreases in CLI (n = 23) and cases (n = 21) were similar, whereas there were fewer decreases among

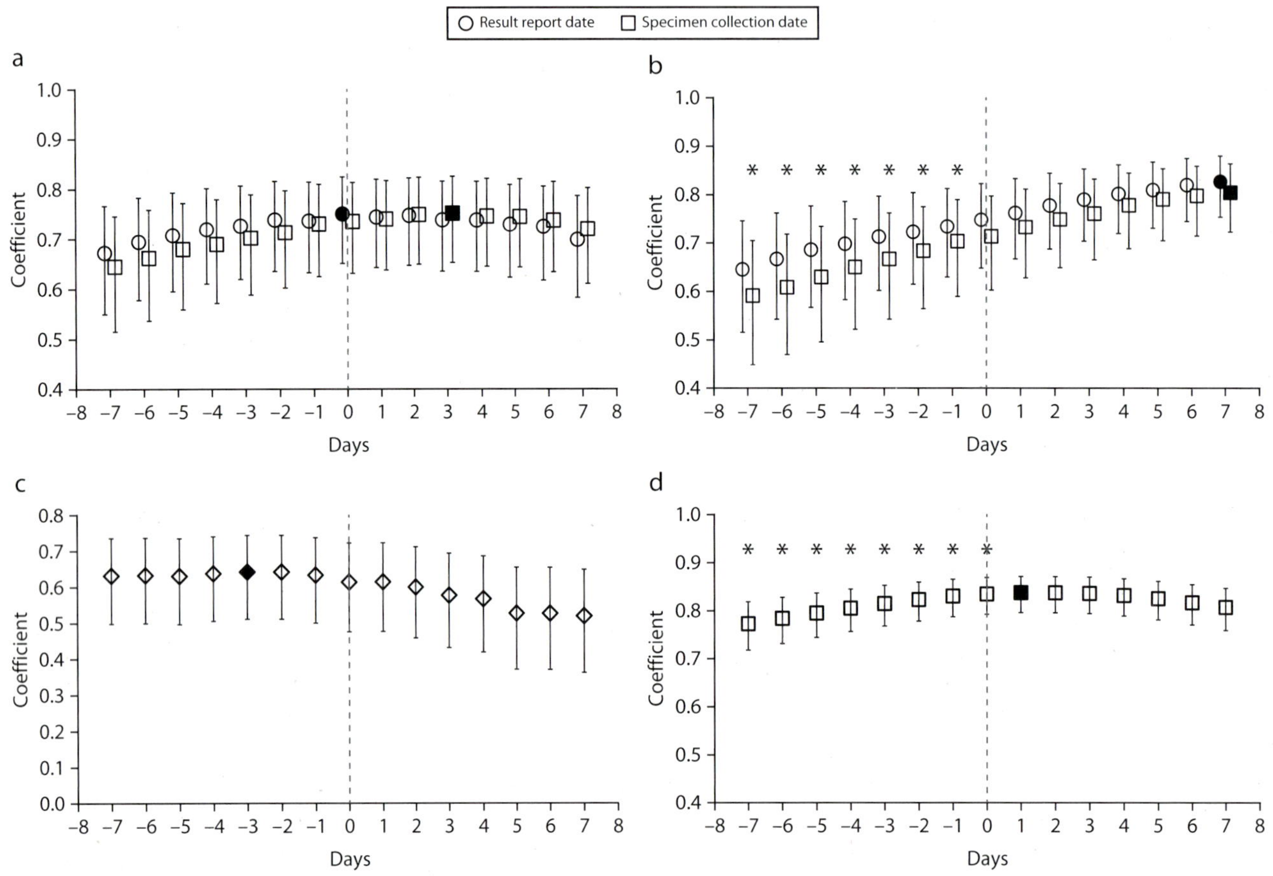

FIGURE 3— **Spearman's Rank Correlation Coefficients for Associations Between COVID-19 Surveillance Data Sets Offset Forward or Backward in Time for (a) Lab-Confirmed Cases Offset Relative to Wastewater Influent, (b) Lab-Confirmed Cases Offset Relative to Wastewater Solids, (c) CLI Offset Relative to Wastewater Influent, and (d) Lab-Confirmed Cases Offset Relative to CLI: Raleigh, NC, Sewershed, April 10–December 13, 2020**

Note. CLI = COVID-like illness. Filled-in markers indicate maximum coefficients. Asterisks indicate coefficients significantly different from the maximum after Bonferroni adjustment (the specimen collection date was used for case significance testing) according to bootstrap analyses of the distribution of coefficients ($P < .05$).

wastewater solids (n = 15) and wastewater influent (n = 9).

Trend Agreement Across Surveillance Data Sets

There were 9 periods for which all data sets agreed with respect to classification of sustained trends: the periods ending June 11, July 2, July 7, July 9, July 11, and November 14 exhibited increasing trends, and the periods ending August 1, September 12, and September 15 exhibited decreasing trends (Figure 4). Not surprisingly, there were no short-term trends that agreed across the 4 surveillance data sets given the temporal shifting of the different surveillance metrics. The wastewater influent and primary solids data sets were in similar agreement with respect to sustained increases when each were compared with lab-confirmed cases.

Specifically, 14 of 51 (27%) increases in cases were also increases in influent data; 16 of the 51 (31%) were increases in solids data. Five of 17 (29%) decreasing trends in case data were decreasing trends according to influent data, whereas 3 (18%) were decreases according to solids data. There was better agreement between lab-confirmed case and CLI data in sustained increases and decreases. Thirty-six of 51 (71%) sustained increases in case data were also sustained increases in CLI data, and 18 of 21 (86%) decreases in case data were also decreases in CLI data.

DISCUSSION

On the day wastewater sample collection began (April 10, 2020), there had been 206 cumulative cases and 41 new cases reported in the sewershed, although the true number of infections is unknown (Figure 1). The Raleigh sewershed had detectable levels of

AJPH January 2023, Vol 113, No. 1

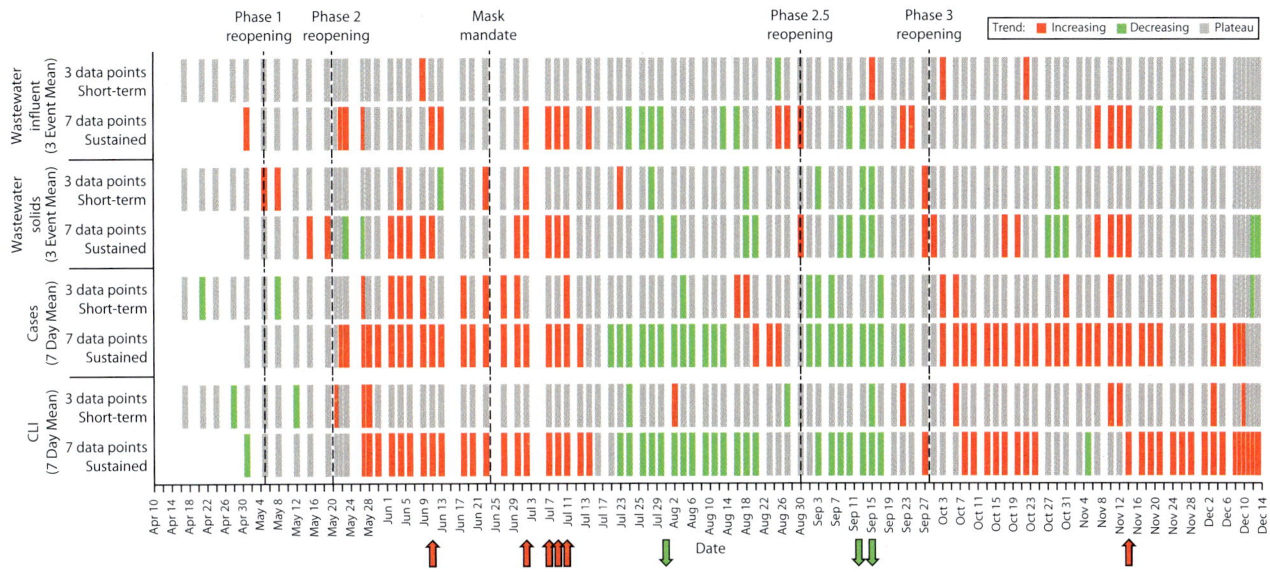

FIGURE 4— Linear Regression Rolling Trend Classifications Illustrating Short-Term (Approximately 1 Week) and Sustained (Approximately 2 Weeks) Trends: Raleigh, NC, Sewershed, April 10–December 13, 2020

Note. CLI = COVID-like illness. Data were smoothed via rolling 7-day averages for cases and CLI and via 3-sampling-event averages for wastewater influent and solids. Statistically significant ($P < .05$) trends are shown in red (increasing) or green (decreasing). Color is placed on the last day of the 3- or 7-point period used in the regression. For lab-confirmed cases, specimen collection date was used. Arrows indicate periods of sustained trends for which there was agreement across the 4 surveillance data sets: the periods ending June 11, July 2, July 7, July 9, July 11, and November 14 (increases; red arrows) and the periods ending August 1, September 12, and September 15 (decreases; green arrows).

SARS-CoV-2 RNA in primary solids in early April, 1 month after the first lab-confirmed COVID-19 case was reported in the sewershed (March 9, 2020). Detection frequency across solids samples was high, as others have reported,[28] despite the fact that primary solids in the Raleigh system also contained waste-activated solids. Monitoring wastewater primary solids was marginally more sensitive than monitoring influent.

SARS-CoV-2 RNA levels in wastewater influent were highly correlated with lab-confirmed cases, as has been reported for other wastewater–case comparisons.[7,20] Despite the longer solids residence time in primary clarifiers, RNA concentrations in primary solids were also correlated highly with lab-confirmed cases, as others have reported.[7,28,29]

CLI being correlated with both measures of wastewater surveillance is notable given that CLI–wastewater agreement has not been widely investigated. Case or CLI correlations with wastewater becoming substantially lower later in the study period (Table B) may have been related to increasing noise in the wastewater signal. As the pandemic progressed, increases in wastewater RNA concentrations from new COVID-19 infections would have occurred in the presence of RNA contributed by individuals who were no longer test positive but continued to shed RNA in feces[30] and residual RNA in the wastewater system.[31,32] In addition, more individuals may have traveled in and out of the sewershed after reopening of public facilities, contributing to greater measurement error in COVID-19 burden based on wastewater.

The strongest correlations observed were between lab-confirmed cases and CLI, even early in the pandemic when there was limited test access and fewer ED visits. Although fewer ED visits would have limited the sensitivity of CLI surveillance for ascertaining infections, CLI may still have strongly correlated with lab-confirmed cases because of a larger overlap in the populations captured by diagnostic testing and CLI surveillance systems. Early in the pandemic, more testing may have been done on individuals who had severe COVID-19 and went to the ED. Noteworthy differences in case and CLI time series occurred later in the study period. A prominent peak in lab-confirmed cases in late August 2020 was not as pronounced in CLI data.

Furthermore, the extent to which cases in December 2020 exceeded previous case peaks in July and August 2020 was not represented in the other surveillance data sets and may reflect increased test access or increased testing around the winter holidays.[4] Widespread

COVID-19 vaccinations or a change in the predominant SARS-CoV-2 variant may affect correlations between different surveillance systems if, for example, the asymptomatic rate increases[33] or the fecal shedding profile is altered.[18] With COVID-19 vaccines now being widely available, wastewater surveillance can be used to identify locations where viral fecal shedding into wastewater is not declining, indicating specific locations of infection.[34]

Multiple surveillance metrics are used in real time by public health officials to provide a fuller COVID-19 public health picture. As such, a temporal comparison is important for the interpretation of agreement or disagreement across surveillance data sets. The reported lead time for wastewater has ranged from 0 to 2 days[8,29] to as high as 2[35] and 3[36,37] weeks. In the Raleigh sewershed, trends in wastewater influent were observed earlier than lab-confirmed case trends when case results report date was used but not when specimen collection date was used, underlining that the potential for wastewater surveillance to provide an earlier warning than clinical testing depends on when test results are reported.[38] The current increased availability of testing and faster turnaround times for case reporting and wastewater surveillance[38] relative to the study period in 2020 may further impact temporal alignment.

Wastewater solids lagged wastewater influent likely because of long solids storage times in Neuse River Resource Recovery Facility primary clarifiers. Wastewater treatment plant design and operation is aimed at wastewater conveyance and treatment and, as such, may not provide ideal conditions for COVID-19 public health surveillance.[39] Therefore, in interpreting wastewater surveillance results, the operation of the facility (with increased communication between plant operators and public health agencies) must be considered.[40] Although the maximum correlation coefficient indicated that rises in CLI were a day behind rises in lab-confirmed cases, syndromic surveillance can be more timely than clinical case surveillance depending on how syndromic data are captured.[41]

The greater numbers of significant trends in lab-confirmed case and CLI metrics than with wastewater metrics indicated a need for public health action at times when wastewater surveillance data did not exhibit a significant change. A limiting factor for numbers of significant trends in wastewater data sets was the 95% statistical confidence requirement for trend classification, which the Centers for Disease Control and Prevention originally recommended but no longer strictly recommends for wastewater surveillance trend reporting.[42] SARS-CoV-2 RNA levels in wastewater primary solids may have had less variability than influent levels as evidenced by the minimal increase in correlation between solids and rolling 7-day average of cases when crude solids data were smoothed (Table A). Therefore, solids surveillance was able to meet the statistical confidence requirement more often than influent surveillance.

PUBLIC HEALTH IMPLICATIONS

We captured COVID-19 dynamics in a major metropolitan area during the first and second waves of infections in 2020. To our knowledge, our study is the first to report agreement between CLI and wastewater surveillance and to demonstrate relationships between key COVID-19 metrics in NC.[43] This study from early in the COVID-19 pandemic, when reportable testing data were better correlated with true disease incidence, supports the use of wastewater and CLI surveillance to complement lab-confirmed case surveillance, especially at times when clinical test penetration is low. AJPH

ABOUT THE AUTHORS

Nadine Kotlarz and Jane A. Hoppin are with the Department of Biological Sciences, North Carolina State University, Raleigh. David A. Holcomb and Lawrence S. Engel are with the Department of Epidemiology, Gillings School of Global Public Health, University of North Carolina, Chapel Hill. A. B. M. Tanvir Pasha, Judith Kays, Yi-Chun Lai, Sean Daly, Francis L. de los Reyes III, and Angela Harris are with the Department of Civil, Construction, and Environmental Engineering, North Carolina State University. Stacie Reckling and Helena Mitasova are with the Center for Geospatial Analytics, North Carolina State University. Sivaranjani Palani is with the Department of Plant and Microbial Biology, North Carolina State University. Erika Bailey is with Raleigh Water, Raleigh, NC. Virginia T. Guidry, Ariel Christensen, and Steven Berkowitz are with the Division of Public Health, North Carolina Department of Health and Human Services, Raleigh.

CORRESPONDENCE

Correspondence should be sent to Nadine Kotlarz, PhD, Department of Biological Sciences, North Carolina State University, 850 Main Campus Dr, Raleigh, NC 27606 (e-mail: nkotlar@ncsu.edu) and Angela Harris, PhD, Department of Civil, Construction, and Environmental Engineering, North Carolina State University, 915 Partners Way, Raleigh, NC, 27606 (e-mail: aharris5@ncsu.edu). Reprints can be ordered at http://www.ajph.org by clicking the "Reprints" link.

PUBLICATION INFORMATION

Full Citation: Kotlarz N, Holcomb DA, Pasha ABMT, et al. Timing and trends for municipal wastewater, lab-confirmed case, and syndromic case surveillance of COVID-19 in Raleigh, North Carolina. *Am J Public Health*. 2023;113(1):79–88.

Acceptance Date: August 26, 2022.

DOI: https://doi.org/10.2105/AJPH.2022.307108

CONTRIBUTORS

N. Kotlarz, F.L. de los Reyes III, and A. Harris contributed to conceptualization and funding acquisition. N. Kotlarz, D.A. Holcomb, E. Bailey, V.T. Guidry, A. Christensen, S. Berkowitz, L.S. Engel, F.L. de los Reyes III, and A. Harris contributed to methodology and resources. N. Kotlarz, A.B.M.T. Pasha, J. Kays, Y.-C. Lai, S. Daly, and S. Palani contributed to investigation. N. Kotlarz, D.A. Holcomb, and S. Reckling contributed to data curation and formal analysis. N.

Kotlarz, D. A. Holcomb, A. B. M. T. Pasha, and S Daly contributed to writing and visualization. N. Kotlarz, D. A. Holcomb, V. Guidry, A. Christensen, S. Berkowitz, J. A. Hoppin, H. Mitasova, L. S. Engel, F. L. de los Reyes III, and A. Harris contributed to writing, review, and editing.

ACKNOWLEDGMENTS

This work was supported by National Science Foundation Rapid Response Research grant CBET- 2029025, the North Carolina Policy Collaboratory, and North Carolina State Center for Human Health and the Environment grant P30ES025128. David A. Holcomb was funded in part by the National Institute of Environmental Health Sciences (grant T32ES007018).

We thank Nathan Howell, Jeremy Lowe, Daniel Cockson, Emma Bolden, Victoria Ponthier, Zach Bennett, Laura Gomez, Ramya Balasubramanian, Marc Serre, Kelly Hoffman, Jeseth Delgado Vela, Adam Smith, Lauren Stadler, Krista Wigginton, Eric Johnson, and Aaron Fleischauer for their contributions to this work.

CONFLICTS OF INTEREST

There are no known potential or actual conflicts of interest.

HUMAN PARTICIPANT PROTECTION

The use of North Carolina Department of Health and Human Services health tracking data was approved by the University of North Carolina institutional review board. Because this was a secondary analysis of de-identified data collected for administrative purposes, it was not necessary or possible to obtain informed consent.

REFERENCES

1. North Carolina Department of Health and Human Services. NCDHHS communicable disease surveillance and reporting. Available at: https://epi.dph.ncdhhs.gov/cd/report.html. Accessed November 15, 2021.
2. Hart OE, Halden RU. Computational analysis of SARS-CoV-2/COVID-19 surveillance by wastewater-based epidemiology locally and globally: feasibility, economy, opportunities and challenges. *Sci Total Environ.* 2020;730:138875. https://doi.org/10.1016/j.scitotenv.2020.138875
3. Vogels CB, Brito AF, Wyllie AL, et al. Analytical sensitivity and efficiency comparisons of SARS-CoV-2 RT–qPCR primer–probe sets. *Nat Microbiol.* 2020;5(10):1299–1305. https://doi.org/10.1038/s41564-020-0761-6
4. Centers for Disease Control and Prevention. Previous U.S. viral testing data. Available at: https://www.cdc.gov/coronavirus/2019-ncov/cases-updates/previous-testing-in-us.html. Accessed June 9, 2022.
5. Rader B, Gertz A, Iuliano AD, et al. Use of at-home COVID-19 tests—United States, August 23, 2021–March 12, 2022. *MMWR Morb Mortal Wkly Rep.* 2022;71(13):489. https://doi.org/10.15585/mmwr.mm7113e1
6. Kirby AE, Walters MS, Jennings WC, et al. Using wastewater surveillance data to support the COVID-19 response—United States, 2020–2021. *MMWR Morb Mortal Wkly Rep.* 2021;70(36):1242–1244. https://doi.org/10.15585/mmwr.mm7036a2
7. Graham KE, Loeb SK, Wolfe MK, et al. SARS-CoV-2 RNA in wastewater settled solids is associated with COVID-19 cases in a large urban sewershed. Available at: https://www.ncbi.nlm.nih.gov/pmc/articles/PMC7737534. Accessed June 9, 2022.
8. Peccia J, Zulli A, Brackney DE, et al. Measurement of SARS-CoV-2 RNA in wastewater tracks community infection dynamics. *Nat Biotechnol.* 2020;38(10):1164–1167. https://doi.org/10.1038/s41587-020-0684-z
9. Centers for Disease Control and Prevention. Public health interpretation and use of wastewater surveillance data. Available at: https://www.cdc.gov/healthywater/surveillance/wastewater-surveillance/public-health-interpretation.html. Accessed June 21, 2022.
10. North Carolina Department of Health and Human Services. Electronic health records promoting interoperability/meaningful use requirements. Available at: https://epi.dph.ncdhhs.gov/cd/meaningful_use/syndromic.html. Accessed June 22, 2022.
11. Cavany S, Bivins A, Wu Z, et al. Inferring SARS-CoV-2 RNA shedding into wastewater relative to the time of infection. *Epidemiol Infect.* 2022;150:e21.
12. Randazzo W, Truchado P, Cuevas-Ferrando E, Simón P, Allende A, Sánchez G. SARS-CoV-2 RNA in wastewater anticipated COVID-19 occurrence in a low prevalence area. *Water Res.* 2020;181:115942. https://doi.org/10.1016/j.watres.2020.115942
13. Waller AE, Scholer M, Ising AI, Travers DA. Using emergency department data for biosurveillance: the North Carolina experience. Available at: https://www.ncbi.nlm.nih.gov/pmc/articles/PMC7120837. Accessed June 22, 2022.
14. Toronto Water. Ashbridges Bay Wastewater Treatment Plant 2017 annual report. Available at: https://www.toronto.ca/wp-content/uploads/2018/05/8e4a-2017-TAB-Annual-Report-Final.pdf. Accessed June 22, 2022.
15. XCG Consultants Ltd. Water and energy conservation guidance manual for sewage works. Available at: https://www.ontario.ca/document/water-and-energy-conservation-guidance-manual-sewage-works-0. Accessed June 22, 2022.
16. Centers for Disease Control and Prevention. Wastewater surveillance testing methods. Available at: https://www.cdc.gov/healthywater/surveillance/wastewater-surveillance/testing-methods.html. Accessed June 10, 2022.
17. North Carolina Department of Health and Human Services. NCDHHS emergency department syndrome definitions. Available at: https://ncdetect.org/case-definitions. Accessed December 10, 2021.
18. Bivins A, Bibby K. Wastewater surveillance during mass COVID-19 vaccination on a college campus. *Environ Sci Technol Lett.* 2021;8(9):792–798. https://doi.org/10.1021/acs.estlett.1c00519
19. D'Aoust PM, Graber TE, Mercier E, et al. Catching a resurgence: increase in SARS-CoV-2 viral RNA identified in wastewater 48 h before COVID-19 clinical tests and 96 h before hospitalizations. *Sci Total Environ.* 2021;770:145319. https://doi.org/10.1016/j.scitotenv.2021.145319
20. Feng S, Roguet A, McClary-Gutierrez JS, et al. Evaluation of sampling, analysis, and normalization methods for SARS-CoV-2 concentrations in wastewater to assess COVID-19 burdens in Wisconsin communities. Available at: https://pubs.acs.org/doi/10.1021/acsestwater.1c00160. Accessed December 10, 2021.
21. Larsen DA, Collins MB, Du Q, et al. Coupling freedom from disease principles and early warning from wastewater surveillance to improve health security. *PNAS Nexus.* 2022;1(1):pgac001. https://doi.org/10.1093/pnasnexus/pgac001
22. Maharaj AS, Parker J, Hopkins JP, et al. Comparison of longitudinal trends in self-reported symptoms and COVID-19 case activity in Ontario, Canada. *PLoS One.* 2022;17(1):e0262447. https://doi.org/10.1371/journal.pone.0262447
23. Wilcox RR. Comparing Pearson correlations: dealing with heteroscedasticity and nonnormality. *Commun Stat Simul Comput.* 2009;38(10):2220–2234. https://doi.org/10.1080/03610910903289151
24. Wilcox RR. *Introduction to Robust Estimation and Hypothesis Testing.* New York, NY: Academic Press; 2011.
25. Gasparrini A, Armstrong B, Kenward MG. Distributed lag non-linear models. *Stat Med.* 2010;29(21):2224–2234. https://doi.org/10.1002/sim.3940
26. Government of North Carolina. North Carolina introduces COVID-19 county alert system. Available at: https://governor.nc.gov/news/press-releases/2020/11/17/north-carolina-introduces-covid-19-county-alert-system. Accessed June 22, 2022.
27. Centers for Disease Control and Prevention. National Wastewater Surveillance System. Available at: https://www.cdc.gov/coronavirus/2019-ncov/cases-updates/wastewater-surveillance.html. Accessed January 7, 2021.
28. Wolfe MK, Topol A, Knudson A, et al. High-frequency, high-throughput quantification of SARS-CoV-2 RNA in wastewater settled solids at eight publicly owned treatment works in northern California shows strong association with COVID-19 incidence. *mSystems.* 2021;6(5):e0082921. https://doi.org/10.1128/mSystems.00829-21
29. D'Aoust PM, Mercier E, Montpetit D, et al. Quantitative analysis of SARS-CoV-2 RNA from wastewater solids in communities with low COVID-19 incidence and prevalence. *Water Res.* 2021;188:116560. https://doi.org/10.1016/j.watres.2020.116560
30. Chen Y, Chen L, Deng Q, et al. The presence of SARS-CoV-2 RNA in the feces of COVID-19 patients. *J Med Virol.* 2020;92(7):833–840. https://doi.org/10.1002/jmv.25825
31. Yang S, Dong Q, Li S, et al. Persistence of SARS-CoV-2 RNA in wastewater after the end of the COVID-19 epidemics. *J Hazard Mater.* 2022;429:128358. https://doi.org/10.1016/j.jhazmat.2022.128358
32. Morales Medina WR, D'Elia S, Fahrenfeld NL. Accumulation of SARS-CoV-2 RNA in sewer biofilms. *ACS EST Water.* 2022; Epub ahead of print. https://doi.org/10.1021/acsestwater.1c00345
33. Bernal JL, Andrews N, Gower C, et al. Effectiveness of the Pfizer-BioNTech and Oxford-AstraZeneca vaccines on Covid-19 related symptoms, hospital admissions, and mortality in older adults in England: test negative case-control study. *BMJ.* 2021;373:n1088. https://doi.org/10.1136/bmj.n1088
34. Smith T, Cassell G, Bhatnagar A. Wastewater surveillance can have a second act in COVID-19

vaccine distribution. Available at: https://jamanetwork.com/journals/jama-health-forum/fullarticle/2775225. Accessed January 7, 2021.

35. Kumar M, Joshi M, Patel AK, Joshi CG. Unravelling the early warning capability of wastewater surveillance for COVID-19: a temporal study on SARS-CoV-2 RNA detection and need for the escalation. *Environ Res.* 2021;196:110946. https://doi.org/10.1016/j.envres.2021.110946

36. Ahmed W, Tscharke B, Bertsch PM, et al. SARS-CoV-2 RNA monitoring in wastewater as a potential early warning system for COVID-19 transmission in the community: a temporal case study. *Sci Total Environ.* 2021;761:144216. https://doi.org/10.1016/j.scitotenv.2020.144216

37. Karthikeyan S, Nguyen A, McDonald D, et al. Rapid, large-scale wastewater surveillance and automated reporting system enable early detection of nearly 85% of COVID-19 cases on a university campus. *mSystems.* 2021;6(4):e0079321. https://doi.org/10.1128/mSystems.00793-21

38. Bibby K, Bivins A, Wu Z, North D. Making waves: plausible lead time for wastewater based epidemiology as an early warning system for COVID-19. *Water Res.* 2021;202:117438. https://doi.org/10.1016/j.watres.2021.117438

39. Medema G, Been F, Heijnen L, Petterson S. Implementation of environmental surveillance for SARS-CoV-2 virus to support public health decisions: opportunities and challenges. *Curr Opin Environ Sci Health.* 2020;17:49–71. https://doi.org/10.1016/j.coesh.2020.09.006

40. McClary-Gutierrez JS, Mattioli MC, Marcenac P, et al. SARS-CoV-2 wastewater surveillance for public health action. *Emerg Infect Dis.* 2021;27(9):1–8. https://doi.org/10.3201/eid2709.210753

41. Maharaj AS, Parker J, Hopkins JP, et al. Anticipating the curve: can online symptom-based data reflect COVID-19 case activity in Ontario. Available at: https://www.medrxiv.org/content/10.1101/2021.01.15.21249879v1.full.pdf. Accessed January 7, 2021.

42. Centers for Disease Control and Prevention. Wastewater surveillance data reporting and analytics. Available at: https://www.cdc.gov/coronavirus/2019-ncov/cases-updates/wastewater-surveillance/data-reporting-analytics.html. Accessed February 4, 2021.

43. North Carolina Department of Health and Human Services. North Carolina COVID-19 Dashboard. Available at: https://covid19.ncdhhs.gov/dashboard. Accessed June 10, 2022.

Effect of the COVID-19 Global Pandemic on Illinois Children Tested for Blood Lead Level and Exposure

Frida D. Fokum, PhD, MS, Tara Entezar, BS, and Kert McAfee, BS

Objectives. To determine whether the number of children tested for lead exposure and the number of case rates increased (rate ratio [RR] > 1), decreased (RR < 1), or remained stable (RR = 1) during COVID-19 pandemic year 2020 compared with prepandemic year 2019.

Methods. We analyzed more than 415 000 children's records reported to the Illinois Department of Public Health in 2019 and 2020 by demographic characteristics. The testing rate was the number of children tested yearly per population. The case rate was the proportion of children whose yearly tests showed a blood lead level of 5 or more micrograms per deciliter. RR was the 2020 case rate divided by the 2019 case rate.

Results. In 2020, 19.6% of children were tested for lead compared with 25.5% in 2019. Testing decreased in 97% of counties. The 24% decreased testing in 2020 was notably in African Americans (36.4% decrease), high-risk zip codes (29.8% decrease), and rural counties (26.9% decrease). Case rates increased in rural counties, high-risk zip codes, Whites, and Hispanics.

Conclusions. During pandemic year 2020, the number of children tested for lead decreased by 24%, and case rates increased in 51% of counties.

Public Health Implications. Redesignation of high-risk zip codes is recommended to increase the testing of at-risk populations. (*Am J Public Health*. 2023;113(1):89–95. https://doi.org/10.2105/AJPH.2022.307109)

AJPH January 2023, Vol 113, No. 1

Lead is a neurotoxin,[1] and there is no safe level of lead in the body. Lead exposure is one of the most prevalent, yet preventable environmental health hazards and can affect any family regardless of socioeconomic status. The damaging health effects lead exposure causes are irreversible. Childhood lead exposure contributes to learning disabilities, developmental delays, and behavioral problems.[2] The percentage of Illinois children whose tests showed lead in their blood remains among the highest in the nation.[3] The mission of the Illinois Lead Program is to eliminate lead exposure. One goal of the Illinois Lead Program is to identify children exposed to lead and provide prompt interventions to improve health and developmental outcomes.[4] Only a blood test can ascertain exposure to lead. Illinois law requires that all blood lead tests be reported to the Illinois Department of Public Health (IDPH).[5] In 2019, Illinois adopted a blood lead level (BLL) of 5 or more micrograms per deciliter (µg/dL) as the new public health intervention level. Intervention is initiated when a BLL of 5 or more µg/dL is confirmed via venipuncture.[5]

On March 11, 2020, the World Health Organization declared COVID-19—with its potential for causing severe respiratory distress, fever, and cough, which could be fatal—a global pandemic.[6,7] Stay-at-home orders and social distance mitigations were implemented statewide to reduce multiplication of the virus.[8] As COVID-19 spread, multiple levels and phases of public health interventions likely influenced lead testing across 2020.

The Centers for Disease Control and Prevention (CDC) reported that, throughout the United States, fewer children were tested for lead exposure in the months following the declaration of the COVID-19 pandemic than in 2019.[9] However, the CDC report did not include the effect of the pandemic on the proportion of children whose tests demonstrated BLLs high enough to qualify for public health intervention (i.e., case rates) or these children's demographic characteristics.

We sought to determine whether the number of children tested and the proportion of tested children with confirmed BLLs of 5 or more μg/dL (case rates) increased, decreased, or remained stable during the COVID-19 pandemic year of 2020 compared with the prepandemic year 2019 among children younger than 6 years at time of blood test, by selected demographic characteristics.

METHODS

Illinois adapted the CDC-sponsored, Healthy Housing and Lead Poisoning Surveillance System as its blood lead–tracking application and management platform in 2017. This centralized Web-based system provides direct access to blood lead test results and collaboration between the IDPH and local health departments around the state. The structured query language system provides tools for the Illinois Lead Program to track and manage blood lead surveillance, testing location, environmental investigations, abatement, mitigation, and case management activities.[10]

Blood Lead Tests

We analyzed more than 415 000 blood lead tests that had been reported to the IDPH of children younger than 6 years that were collected between January 2019 and December 2020 in Illinois. Blood lead is collected via venous (venipuncture) or capillary (fingerstick) methodology. Hospitals, local health departments, laboratories, and medical professionals perform blood lead analyses and evaluate, diagnose, and treat lead-exposed children. A capillary BLL of 5 or more μg/dL is required to be confirmed with a venipuncture draw sent to a certified reference laboratory. Public health intervention was initiated when a child tested positive with a BLL of 5 or more μg/dL.

Illinois law requires all licensed, registered, or approved health care facility serving children younger than 6 years to ensure that children are evaluated for risk, tested for lead exposure, or both.[5] Furthermore, health care providers, hospital administrators, public health officers, and directors of clinical laboratories who have verified information of the existence of a blood lead test result for any child must report the result to the IDPH.

Illinois law requires any BLL of 5 or more μg/dL to be reported to the IDPH within 48 hours after analysis. All other blood lead test results (< 5 μg/dL) must be reported to the IDPH no later than 30 days following the last day of the month in which the test results were analyzed.[5]

All children younger than 6 years are required to be evaluated for lead exposure risks by their physician and tested if necessary. Illinois recommends that all children be evaluated or tested as indicated at ages 12 and 24 months and 3, 4, 5, and 6 years according to the Childhood Lead Risk Questionnaire.[11] The case manager assigned to the child's case, along with the medical provider, should discuss the importance of regular blood lead testing and continue to monitor the child's follow-up BLLs. The recommended follow-up schedule for repeat testing ranges from within 1 week for BLL of 45 or more μg/dL to 3 months for BLL of 5 to 14 μg/dL.[11] State and federal mandates require all children enrolled in Medicaid programs to be tested for lead exposure regardless of where they live.[12,13]

Rural and Urban Areas

Of the 102 Illinois counties, 83 are predominantly rural. Rural areas are not part of a metropolitan statistical area or are part of a metropolitan statistical area with a population of less than 60 000.[14,15] Urban areas include 18 counties and the city of Chicago, where 22% of Illinois children reside.

High-Risk Zip Codes

Illinois law requires the IDPH to designate areas of the state where children are at highest risk for lead exposure.[5] Of Illinois' more than 1500 zip codes, 581 are designated as high risk so they have mandated lead testing requirements. High-risk zip codes are designated based on socioeconomic status and proportion of pre-1978 housing units with lead-based paint prevalence or hazards.[16] We obtained the number of pre-1978 housing units from US Census 2020 data.[14] We adapted the prevalence of lead in housing units from the American Healthy Homes Survey.[17]

Data Analyses

We conducted a retrospective comparative analysis of children tested for blood lead during prepandemic year 2019 and pandemic year 2020, stratified by demographic characteristics. We determined that changes in the number of children tested, testing rates, case rates, and rate ratios (RRs) occurred from all childhood blood lead records reported to the IDPH. We calculated testing rate as the number of children tested for lead in blood yearly (numerator) divided by the population of children according to the US Census 2020 (denominator) expressed as percentages. Case rate refers to the proportion of children tested with a confirmed BLL of 5 or more µg/dL per year. RR expressed as 2020 case rate divided by 2019 case rate indicated an increased (RR > 1), decreased (RR < 1), or stable (RR = 1) case rate in pandemic year 2020 compared with 2019. Illinois law requires that any IDPH release of data to the public be done in aggregate form to eliminate disclosure conflicts with state or federal laws regarding personal health information.[5]

We categorized results by county of residence, rural versus urban county designation, high-risk versus low-risk zip codes for lead exposure, age, sex, race, and ethnicity. Year was a key analytic variable. We counted a child only once in a year if the child had multiple tests. Any capillary BLL of 5 or more µg/dL had to be confirmed through a venous test. We considered only venous BLLs of 5 or more µg/dL as confirmed results for the detection of case rates. We selected the highest venous result per child per year as a confirmatory test. We used the χ^2 test to analyze differences in testing and case rates by categorical variables ($\alpha = 0.05$). We considered $P < .05$ as statistically significant. We conducted the statistical analyses using SAS version 9.4 (SAS Institute, Cary, NC).

RESULTS

We found decreases in the testing rate and the case rate following the declaration of COVID-19 as a global pandemic in 2020.

Number Tested in 2020

A total of 228 614 and 173 204 Illinois children were tested for blood lead in 2019 and 2020, respectively. Among approximately 900 000 children younger than 6 years residing in Illinois, 25.5% were tested for lead in 2019 compared with 19.6% in 2020. Approximately 55 000 fewer children were tested in 2020 than in 2019, indicating a 24% decrease. Testing rate by sex was similar for boys and girls in 2019 and 2020, although approximately 5% more boys are tested on a yearly basis. Based on age, a substantial decrease in testing ranged from 18.5% for children aged 1 year to 33.1% for children aged 4 years. The largest decline in testing rate was recorded for non-Hispanic Black and African American children (36.4%), a nearly 50% higher decrease compared with non-Hispanic White or Latino children (Figure 1a). Sixty-four of the 102 Illinois counties (12.5% of which were urban and 87.5% rural) reported a more than 24% decrease in children tested. The decrease in testing was substantial, particularly in the southern and western parts of Illinois. High-risk zip code areas saw significant declines in testing (29.8%) compared with a 22.9% decrease in the rest of the state. Three of the 102 counties showed increased testing during the pandemic year 2020 (Figure 2).

Case Rates

The number of Illinois children tested with a confirmed BLL of 5 or more µg/dL was 27% less in 2020 than in 2019. The Illinois case rate decreased to 1.7% in pandemic year 2020 compared with 1.8% in 2019. However, case rates increased (RR > 1) in 2020 for children residing in rural counties or high-risk zip codes and for non-Hispanic Whites and Hispanics and Latinos compared with prepandemic year 2019 (Figure 1b). Case rates remained stable (RR = 1) for children residing outside Chicago, children younger than 3 years, and girls. Conversely, case rates decreased (RR < 1) for Illinois as a whole, Chicago, urban counties, low-risk zip codes, boys, children aged 3 or 4 years, Black and African American individuals, and Asians.

At the county level, case rates fluctuated between pandemic and prepandemic periods. In 2020, based on 102 counties of residence, case rates increased (51%), decreased (41%), or remained stable (8%) compared with prepandemic year 2019. Counties with these various shifts were dispersed across the state. Of the 51% counties with increased case rates, 81% were rural and 19% were urban. The 41% of counties with decreased case rates were 83% rural and 17% urban (Figure 2).

DISCUSSION

The results of this work showed a 24% decrease in testing rate and a decrease in overall case rate in pandemic year 2020 compared with prepandemic year 2019.

As previously stated, Illinois law[5] requires physicians licensed to practice medicine in Illinois and health care providers who see or treat children to test those children for lead exposure when they reside in or frequently visit a high-risk area. Children residing in areas the IDPH defines as low risk are evaluated using the Childhood Lead Risk Questionnaire,[11] and if they are determined to be at potential risk for lead exposure, they must receive a blood lead

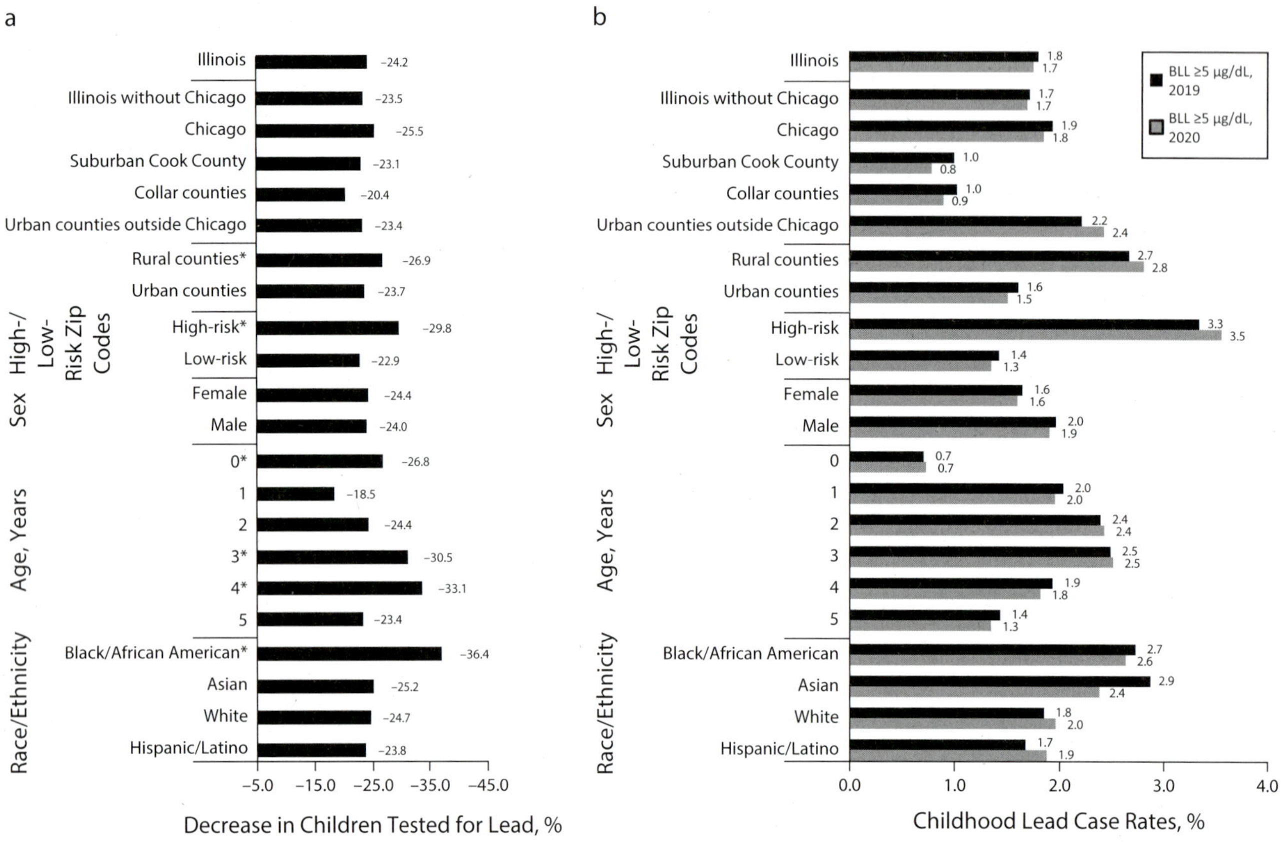

FIGURE 1— Illinois Children Tested for Lead in Blood in Pandemic Year 2020 Compared with Prepandemic Year 2019 by Select Demographics and (a) Decrease in Percentage of Children Tested, and (b) Percentage of Childhood Lead Case Rates

Note. BLL = blood lead level; μg/dL = micrograms per deciliter. Children were younger than 6 years at time of blood test. Testing rate was the number of children tested for blood lead by year (numerator) divided by the population of children per 2020 US Census (denominator). The case rate was the proportion of children tested with confirmed elevated BLL ≥ 5 μg/dL (numerator) divided by children tested by year (denominator, %). In panel b, the percentages listed are rounded.
Source. Illinois Department of Public Health–Healthy Housing and Lead Poisoning Surveillance Data 2019–2020.
*Significant at $P < .05$.

test. This evaluation is to be performed annually during a well-child visit or physical checkup.

Recent trends indicate that blood lead testing has been steadily declining at a rate of 4% nationally.[18] The 24% decrease in the testing rate in 2020 compared with that of 2019 was significant compared with decreases in preceding years. The largest decrease in the number of children tested occurred during the 6 months following the declaration of the COVID-19 pandemic, when the strictest COVID-19 mitigations were in place.[8] Illinois recorded a 38% decrease in testing in those months compared with a 34% decrease nationally per the CDC.[9] In addition to the long-term trend, stay-at-home orders and travel restrictions hindered routine medical care, including testing for elevated BLLs. Also, during the COVID-19 surges in 2020, physicians performed remote medical visits, making lead testing during a well-child visit impossible.

In 1 case, a county with 74% pre-1978 housing units experienced a 46% decrease in the number of children tested during the pandemic. Quarterly reports sent to the IDPH from that county's local health department stated that lead testing decreased during the pandemic because immunization and Special Supplemental Nutrition Program for Women, Infants, and Children clinics were closed. Moreover, collaborations with health care providers and school nurses were limited to telephone interactions.

In February 2019, Illinois adopted a BLL of 5 or more μg/dL as the minimum level requiring the initiation of public health intervention, limiting our study to 2019 and later. Based on environmental inspection findings, the

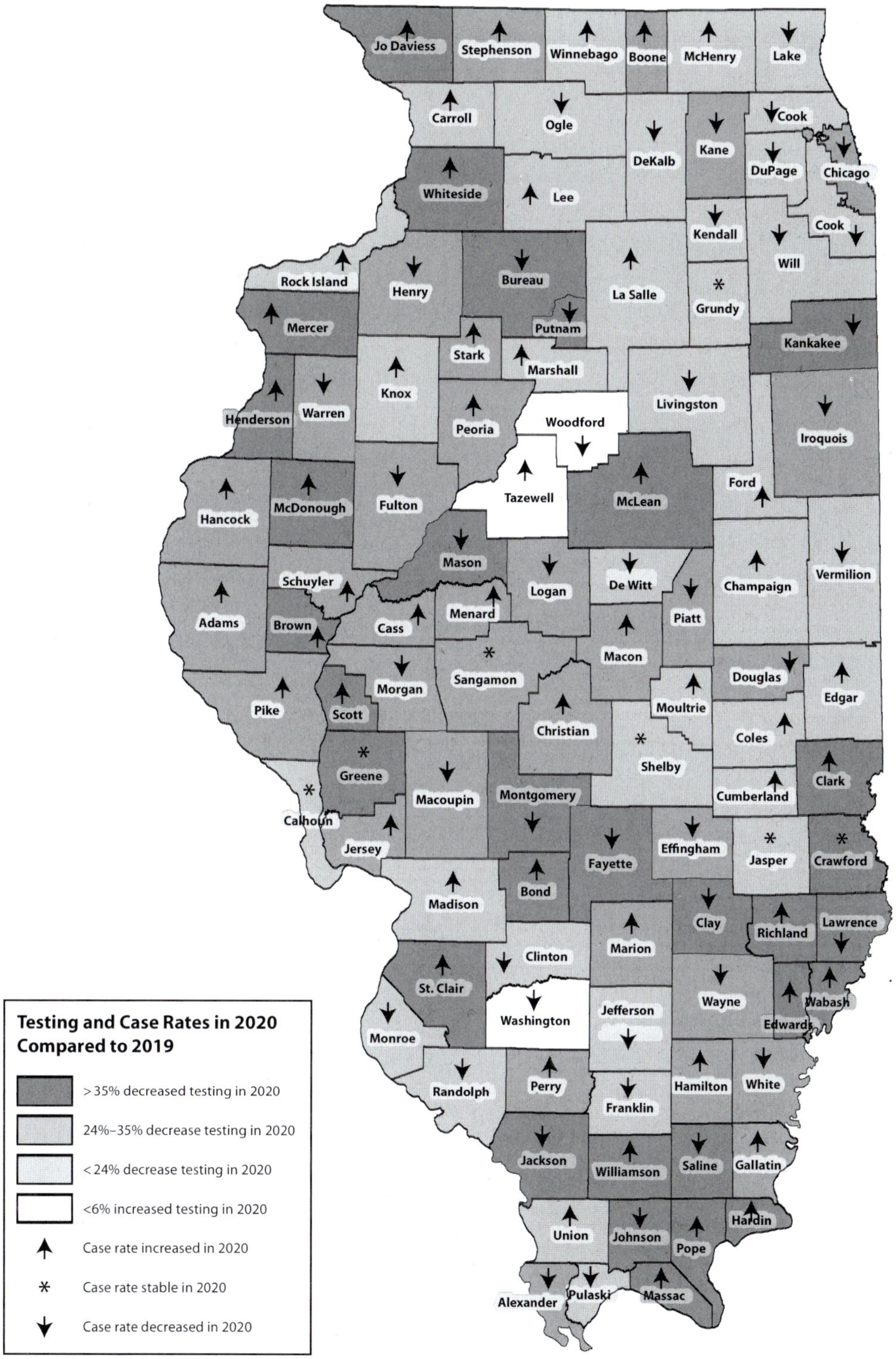

FIGURE 2— Illinois Children Tested for Blood Lead Exposure and Case Rates in Pandemic Year 2020 Compared With Prepandemic Year 2019 by County

Note. BLL = blood lead level; µg/dL = micrograms per deciliter; RR = rate ratio. Children were younger than 6 years at the time of blood testing. Testing rate was the proportion of children tested for blood lead by year (numerator) divided by the population of children per 2020 US Census (denominator, %). Case rate was the percentage of children tested with confirmed lead levels ≥ 5 µg/dL (numerator) divided by children tested by year (denominator). RR or 2020 case rate divided by 2019 case rate increased (RR > 1), decreased (RR < 1), or remained stable (RR = 1).
Source. Illinois Department of Public Health–Healthy Housing and Lead Poisoning Surveillance Data 2019–2020.

most common cause of lead in blood in Illinois children is exposure to lead paint and dust found in older housing. Approximately 65% of the state's housing units were built before 1978, the year lead paint was banned. The *New York Times* described lead exposure as a COVID-19 side effect owing to the lockdown.[19] Children spent more time at home during the pandemic. Some families and homeowners performed home renovations with minimal safety precautions, increasing the risk of lead exposure. However, because of decreased testing, fewer children were identified with lead in blood.

High-risk zip codes are found throughout Illinois, especially in the western portion of the state and a cluster in Cook County. Our most concerning findings were decreased lead testing rates and increased case rates in 52 counties, especially among children residing in designated high-risk zip codes. The risk consideration is that Medicaid-supported children are more likely to live in poorly maintained homes in high-risk zip codes.[12,13]

Our study supports a CDC study that reported a decrease in the number of children tested for blood lead during the COVID-19 pandemic.[9] Additionally, our study expanded on the CDC analysis to include demographic stratifications and case rates. The reduced number of tests and increased case rates may be partially attributable to different populations, as children previously tested with BLLs of less than 5 µg/dL were probably not tested the following year. Children spent more time at home, and most untested children resided in high-risk zip codes. Fewer children were tested for blood lead in pandemic year 2020, and case rates increased in children residing in rural counties or high-risk zip codes and among non-Hispanic White and Hispanic children.

Limitations

We used only BLLs of 5 or more µg/dL obtained by venipuncture to compute case rates. Many providers use LeadCare II point-of-care analyzers to test using finger-stick blood draws. In July 2021, Magellan recalled LeadCare II analytical components manufactured between October 2020 and June 2021 because of the potential for false-negative results.[20] Children whose blood was analyzed with LeadCare II units during the last 3 months of 2020 may have obtained a false-negative diagnosis, resulting in underestimated case rates for 2020.

Public Health Implications

In addition to elimination strategies and regulations established by the IDPH, reevaluation of high-risk zip codes for lead exposure is recommended for increasing the testing of targeted at-risk populations. Strategies to increase testing could include additional health care providers, enhanced remote medical care, and fortified support of programs with reduced capacity. If there is a policy recommendation for universal testing by age, there needs to be a funding mechanism to ensure that all children receive tests at no charge.

Conclusions

The number of Illinois children tested for blood lead decreased by 24% following the declaration of the COVID-19 global pandemic in 2020. The decreased testing was most marked for African Americans, for those in designated high-risk zip codes, and for those in rural counties. Case rates increased for children residing in rural counties or high-risk zip codes and for non-Hispanic Whites and Hispanics or Latinos compared with prepandemic year 2019. AJPH

ABOUT THE AUTHORS

Frida D. Fokum and Kert McAfee are with the Illinois Department of Public Health, Springfield, IL. Tara Entezar is with the School of Integrative Biology, University of Illinois, Urbana-Champaign.

CORRESPONDENCE

Correspondence should be sent to Kert McAfee, 525 West Jefferson St, Springfield, IL 62761 (e-mail: kert.mcafee@illinois.gov). Reprints can be ordered at http://www.ajph.org by clicking the "Reprints" link.

PUBLICATION INFORMATION

Full Citation: Fokum FD, Entezar T, McAfee K. Effect of the COVID-19 global pandemic on Illinois children tested for blood lead level and exposure. *Am J Public Health*. 2023;113(1):89–95.

Acceptance Date: August 29, 2022.

DOI: https://doi.org/10.2105/AJPH.2022.307109

CONTRIBUTORS

F. D. Fokum conceptualized and designed the study and the study methodology, analyzed and interpreted the data, wrote the first draft of the article, and revised the article after reviewer and editor comments. T. Entezar created the map using ArcGIS. T. Entezar and K. McAfee reviewed the first draft of the article. K. McAfee supervised the study and revised and approved the final version of the article.

ACKNOWLEDGMENTS

Funding for the Illinois Lead Program was provided by the Centers for Disease Control and Prevention (grant FAIN-NUE2EH001412), the US Environmental Protection Agency (grant FAIN-00E31611 BG), the Illinois Lead Poisoning Screening, Prevention, and Abatement Fund, and the Illinois State General Revenue Funds.

This research is part of the Illinois Department of Public Health's surveillance project. We thank Gerrin CheekButler, deputy director, Office of Health Protection, and the Illinois Lead Program Team, Andrew Stewart, Darla Hamende, Helen Wright, Cari Roger, Aubrey Dove, Jenn Kennett, and Sai Prahitha Arra (intern), for general review of the report.

Note. The content of this article is solely the responsibility of the authors and does not necessarily represent the official views of the funders.

CONFLICTS OF INTEREST

We have no potential or actual conflicts of interest to disclose.

HUMAN PARTICIPANT PROTECTION

No protocol approval was necessary because we have reported only aggregated data, per Illinois statute.

REFERENCES

1. Canfield RL, Henderson CR Jr, Cory-Slechta DA, Cox C, Jusko TA, Lanphear BP. Intellectual impairment in children with blood lead concentrations below 10 microg per deciliter. *N Engl J Med.* 2003; 348(16):1517–1526. https://doi.org/10.1056/NEJMoa022848
2. Bellinger DC, Needleman HL. Intellectual impairment and blood lead levels. *N Engl J Med.* 2003; 349(5):500–502; author reply 500–502. https://doi.org/10.1056/NEJM200307313490515
3. Centers for Disease Control and Prevention. CDC blood lead levels (μg/DL) among US children < 72 months of age, by state, year, and blood lead level (BLL) group. Available at: https://www.cdc.gov/nceh/lead/docs/cbls-national-data-table-508.pdf. Accessed June 29, 2022.
4. Illinois Department of Public Health. Childhood lead poisoning surveillance. Available at: https://dph.illinois.gov/topics-services/environmental-health-protection/lead-poisoning-prevention/childhood-surveillance.html. Accessed June 29, 2022.
5. Illinois General Assembly. 410 ILCS 45, Lead Poisoning Prevention Act. Available at: https://www.ilga.gov/legislation/ilcs/ilcs3.asp?ActID=1523&ChapterID=35. Accessed June 29, 2022.
6. Cucinotta D, Vanelli M. WHO declares COVID-19 a pandemic. *Acta Biomed.* 2020;91(1):157–160. https://doi.org/10.23750/abm.v91i1.9397
7. Ren LL, Wang YM, Wu ZQ, et al. Identification of a novel coronavirus causing severe pneumonia in human: a descriptive study. *Chin Med J (Engl).* 2020;133(9):1015–1024. https://doi.org/10.1097/CM9.0000000000000722
8. State of Illinois. Executive order in response to COVID-19 (COVID-19 Executive Order no. 8). March 20, 2020. Available at: https://www2.illinois.gov/Documents/ExecOrders/2020/ExecutiveOrder-2020-10.pdf. Accessed June 29, 2022.
9. Centers for Disease Control and Prevention. Decreases in young children who received blood lead level testing during COVID-19—34 jurisdictions, January–May 2020. *MMWR Morb Mortal Wkly Rep.* 2021;70(5):155-161. https://doi.org/10.15585/mmwr.mm7005a2.
10. Centers for Disease Control and Prevention. HHLPSS data management platform. July 30, 2019. Available at: https://www.cdc.gov/nceh/lead/data/hhlpss.htm. Accessed October 30, 2022.
11. State of Illinois. Childhood Lead Risk Questionnaire (CLRQ) algorithm. Available at: https://dph.illinois.gov/content/dam/soi/en/web/idph/files/publications/clrq-algorithm.pdf. Accessed October 30, 2022.
12. Centers for Disease Control and Prevention. Recommendations for blood lead screening of Medicaid-eligible children aged 1–5 years: an updated approach to targeting a group at high risk. *MMWR Recomm Rep.* 2009;58(RR-9):1–11.
13. Illinois Department of Healthcare and Family Services. Provider blood lead screening report. Available at: https://www2.illinois.gov/hfs/MedicalProviders/NonInstitutional/Pages/ProviderBloodLead.aspx. Accessed June 29, 2022.
14. US Census Bureau. American Community Survey 5-year data (2009–2017). December 6, 2018. Available at: https://www.census.gov/data/developers/data-sets/acs-5year.html. Accessed October 30, 2022.
15. Illinois Department of Public Health. Illinois counties by rural/urban classification. Available at: http://www.idph.state.il.us/RuralHealth/Rur_Urb_2021.pdf. Accessed June 29, 2022.
16. Illinois Department of Public Health. Illinois Lead Program: 2015 annual surveillance report. October 2016. Available at: https://dph.illinois.gov/content/dam/soi/en/web/idph/files/publications/lead-surveillance-report-2015-122116.pdf. Accessed June 29, 2022.
17. US Department of Housing and Urban Development. American Healthy Homes Survey II. October 29, 2021. Available at: https://www.hud.gov/sites/dfiles/HH/documents/AHHS_II_Lead_Findings_Report_Final_29oct21.pdf. Accessed June 29, 2022.
18. Wang T, Zhou YP, Sun Y, Zheng YX. Trends in blood lead levels in the US from 1999 to 2016. *Am J Prev Med.* 2021;60(4):e179–e187. https://doi.org/10.1016/j.amepre.2020.10.024
19. Anthes E. More childhood lead poisoning is a side effect of COVID lockdowns. New York Times. March 11, 2021. Available at: https://www.nytimes.com/2021/03/11/health/virus-lead-poisoning-children.html. Accessed June 29, 2022.
20. US Food and Drug Administration. Magellan Diagnostics recalls LeadCare II, LeadCare Plus, and LeadCare Ultra Blood Lead Tests due to risk of falsely low results. March 31, 2022. Available at: https://www.fda.gov/medical-devices/medical-device-recalls/magellan-diagnostics-recalls-leadcare-ii-leadcare-plus-and-leadcare-ultra-blood-lead-tests-due-risk. Accessed June 30, 2022.

SARS-CoV-2 Infection, Hospitalization, and Death in Vaccinated and Infected Individuals by Age Groups in Indiana, 2021–2022

Wanzhu Tu, PhD, Pengyue Zhang, PhD, Anna Roberts, MS, Katie S. Allen, BS, Jennifer Williams, MPH, Peter Embi, MD, and Shaun Grannis, MD, MS

AJPH January 2023, Vol 113, No. 1

Objectives. To assess the effectiveness of vaccine-induced immunity against new infections, all-cause emergency department (ED) and hospital visits, and mortality in Indiana.

Methods. Combining statewide testing and immunization data with patient medical records, we matched individuals who received at least 1 dose of severe acute respiratory syndrome coronavirus 2 (SARS-CoV-2) vaccines with individuals with previous SARS-CoV-2 infection on index date, age, gender, race/ethnicity, zip code, and clinical diagnoses. We compared the cumulative incidence of infection, all-cause ED visits, hospitalizations, and mortality.

Results. We matched 267 847 pairs of individuals. Six months after the index date, the incidence of SARS-CoV-2 infection was significantly higher in vaccine recipients (6.7%) than the previously infected (2.9%). All-cause mortality in the vaccinated, however, was 37% lower than that of the previously infected. The rates of all-cause ED visits and hospitalizations were 24% and 37% lower in the vaccinated than in the previously infected.

Conclusions. The significantly lower rates of all-cause ED visits, hospitalizations, and mortality in the vaccinated highlight the real-world benefits of vaccination. The data raise questions about the wisdom of reliance on natural immunity when safe and effective vaccines are available. (*Am J Public Health*. 2023;113(1):96–104. https://doi.org/10.2105/AJPH.2022.307112)

Strong and consistent evidence shows that mRNA vaccines BNT162b2 and mRNA-1273 and the Janssen vaccine JNJ-78436735 confer considerable protection to fully vaccinated individuals against severe acute respiratory syndrome coronavirus 2 (SARS-CoV-2) infection, severe illnesses requiring hospitalization, and mortality.[1–6] However, vaccine effectiveness is not 100%, and the risk of breakthrough infections remains, especially with newer variants.[7,8] Furthermore, data and opinions diverge on the extent of the waning immunity provided by the mRNA vaccines.[9,10] While a population-based observational study suggested that immunity waned in individuals within 2 months after completing the 2-dose sequence of the BNT162b2 vaccine,[11] a randomized clinical trial showed that 6 months after vaccination, the BNT162b2 vaccine's effectiveness against SARS-CoV-2 infection remained strong at higher than 86%; its effectiveness against the severe disease was 96.7%.[12]

Natural immunity induced by SARS-CoV-2 infection also protects against reinfection. Systematic reviews of immunological evidence suggested that SARS-CoV-2–specific immunity appeared soon after infection.[13,14] Extensive observational studies confirmed the significantly reduced risk for subsequent infection by more than 80% for at least 6 to 12 months in individuals with previous infection.[15–17] Data are mixed on the relative levels of protection conferred by vaccination versus infection.[18–20] Less understood is the real-world time course of the protective effects of previous infection and vaccination against new infection acquisition and all-cause mortality and hospitalization in persons of different age groups. Unlike COVID-19–specific outcomes used by earlier studies, all-cause emergency department (ED) visits, hospitalizations, and mortality cover a broader spectrum of health consequences of the disease.

In this observational cohort study, we leveraged public health immunization data and electronic medical record data from a statewide health information exchange and state health department to examine the incidence rates of SARS-CoV-2 infection, all-cause ED visit, hospitalization, and death in individuals who had been vaccinated compared with those with previous infections in a real-world population.

METHODS

We derived data used in this research from the Indiana Network for Patient Care (INPC), one of the largest health information networks in the United States.[21] Briefly, the INPC is a central repository of clinical and administrative health data from 38 health systems representing 117 hospitals and 18 486 physician practices, commercial laboratories, and public health departments across Indiana. At the emergence of the pandemic, the Indiana Health Information Exchange expanded the INPC system to receive daily feeds of SARS-CoV-2 test results from all statewide testing locations and daily death records through the Indiana State Department of Health and Family Social Services Administration.[22] Furthermore, all COVID-19 vaccine data contained in the Indiana immunization registry were combined with testing and outcomes data.

Study Design

We derived the observational study cohort from the INPC and the Indiana statewide testing data. The cohort consisted of matched pairs of vaccine recipients and unvaccinated individuals with SARS-CoV-2 infections. See Figure A (available as a supplement to the online version of this article at https://ajph.org) for a schematic depiction of the comparison groups. Eligible participants were Indiana residents aged 12 years or older with at least 1 previously recorded health care encounter with the INPC between January 1, 2016, and February 9, 2022; the requirement of a previous encounter ensured a more complete capture of the characteristics of the study participants. Patient medical records in INPC and test data were linked, de-duplicated, and aggregated using a global algorithm.[23] Vaccine data from the state immunization registry were imported into the health information exchange and integrated with laboratory test data.

Observation of infected participants started 30 days after the initial infection and ended at the end of follow-up or vaccination, whichever came first. Similarly, observation of vaccinated participants started 30 days after the initial vaccination and ended with the conclusion of follow-up or infection, whichever came first. We applied the 30-day time window of exclusion to both groups to ensure equal surveillance and comparability.

Matched Cohorts

A vaccine recipient's index date was defined as 30 days after the first SARS-CoV-2 vaccination. In an individual with a previous SARS-CoV-2 infection, we defined the index date as 30 days after the initial infection. In both situations, the initial infection and vaccination represented the first point of viral exposure, whereas the 30-day window approximated the time of immunity development. We matched each vaccine recipient with an infected participant on the index date (+/− 15 days), age, gender, race/ethnicity, zip code, and the number of coexisting conditions that had been identified by the Centers for Disease Control and Prevention (CDC) as "conclusive" or "suggestive" risk factors for severe COVID-19 (https://bit.ly/3gTvA3w; complete lists of CDC-identified comorbid conditions also appear in the footnotes to Table 1). The construction of the matched cohort is depicted in Figure 1.

Outcome Events of Interest

The primary outcome events of interest were SARS-CoV-2 infection in those vaccinated or reinfection for the previously infected participants, all-cause ED visits, hospitalizations, and deaths. All outcome events in the study were identified and extracted from the INPC, and deaths were derived from the State of Indiana death records.

Statistical Analysis

Before comparing the outcome event rates, we examined the balance in demographic and clinical characteristics between the vaccine recipients and infection cases to ensure that the 2 groups were comparable and well matched. We used survival analyses to estimate the cumulative incidence rates of SARS-CoV-2 infection for the vaccinated and reinfection for those with previous infections. We similarly estimated the cumulative rates for hospitalization, ED visit, and death.

TABLE 1— **A Study of SARS-COV-2 Infection, Hospitalizations, and Mortality in Vaccinated and Infected Individuals: Demographic and Clinical Characteristics of the Matched Cohorts on the Index Date, Indiana, 2020–2022**

	Vaccinated (n = 267 847)	Unvaccinated With Previous Infection (n = 267 847)	*P*
Race, no. (%)			> .99
American Indian or Alaska Native	53 (0.0)	53 (0.0)	
Asian/Pacific Islander	1 684 (0.6)	1 684 (0.6)	
Black or African American	21 044 (7.9)	21 044 (7.9)	
Multiracial	43 (0.0)	43 (0.0)	
Other/unknown	9 630 (3.6)	9 630 (3.6)	
White	235 393 (87.9)	235 393 (87.9)	
Ethnicity, no. (%)			< .001
Hispanic or Latino	13 224 (4.9)	16 733 (6.2)	
Not Hispanic or Latino	220 367 (82.3)	235 639 (88.0)	
Other/unknown	34 256 (12.8)	15 475 (5.8)	
Gender, no. (%)			> .99
Female	155 759 (58.2)	155 759 (58.2)	
Male	112 085 (41.8)	112 085 (41.8)	
Unknown	3 (0.0)	3 (0.0)	
Age, y			> .99
Mean (SD)	38.9 (16.4)	38.9 (16.4)	.98
Median (IQR)	37 (26–51)	37 (26–51)	
12–19, no. (%)	31 454 (11.7)	31 454 (11.7)	
20–39, no. (%)	115 511 (43.1)	115 511 (43.1)	
40–59, no. (%)	87 199 (32.5)	87 199 (32.5)	
60–79, no. (%)	31 249 (11.7)	31 249 (11.7)	
80–110, no. (%)	2 434 (0.9)	2 434 (0.9)	
CDC "certain" risk score[a]			
Mean (SD)	0 (0.2)	0 (0.2)	> .99
Median (IQR)	0 (0–0)	0 (0–0)	
CDC "possible" risk score[b]			
Mean (SD)	0.1 (0.3)	0.1 (0.3)	> .99
Median (IQR)	0 (0–0)	0 (0–0)	
CDC sum risk score[c]			
Mean (SD)	0.1 (0.4)	0.1 (0.4)	> .99
Median (IQR)	0 (0–0)	0 (0–0)	

Note. CDC = Centers for Disease Control and Prevention; IQR = interquartile range; SARS-CoV-2 = severe acute respiratory syndrome coronavirus 2.
[a]CDC "certain" risk score conditions: cancer, chronic kidney disease, chronic obstructive pulmonary disease, heart conditions, sickle cell disease, solid organ transplant recipient, type 1 diabetes mellitus, type 2 diabetes mellitus.
[b]CDC "possible" risk score conditions: asthma, cerebrovascular disease, hypertension, immunocompromised state, liver disease, neurologic conditions, obesity, other respiratory diseases, thalassemia.
[c]CDC sum risk score: a sum of how many "certain" and "possible" conditions a person was flagged for.

The index date (i.e., the time zero) represented 30 days after the initial exposure, either to the vaccine or the virus; protection from vaccine-induced and naturally acquired immunity would come after the index date. Matched pairs were censored when an infected participant received a vaccination or a vaccine recipient became infected. Time to mortality that was not observed before the end of the observation window, February 9, 2022, was censored

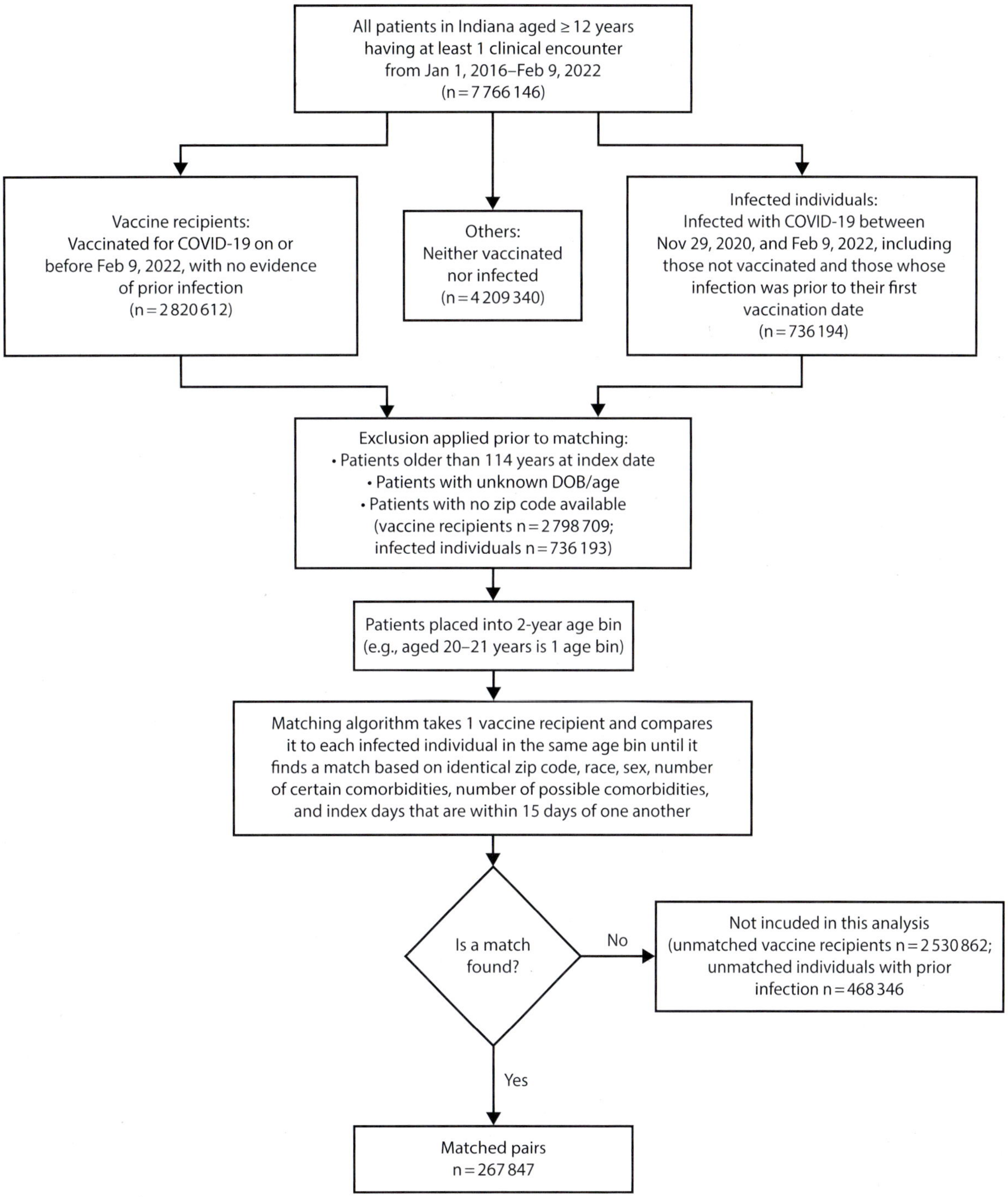

FIGURE 1— Construction of Matched Cohorts of Infected and Vaccinated Individuals: SARS-COV-2 Infection, Hospitalizations, and Mortality in Vaccinated and Infected Individuals, Indiana, 2020–2022

Note. DOB = date of birth; SARS-CoV-2 = severe acute respiratory syndrome coronavirus 2.

(i.e., the patient was alive at the conclusion of the observation period). Time to infection or reinfection, ED visits, and hospitalization was censored at the time of the event, at the end of the observation window, or when the matched individual was censored, whichever came first. For vaccine recipients and individuals with previous infection, we computed the times from the index date to the outcome events or censoring. Cumulative incidence rates were calculated as $1-\hat{S}(t)$, where $\hat{S}(t)$ is the estimated survival function. We used the log-rank test to perform comparisons of the cumulative incidence rates.

We conducted all analyses with R software version 4.1.2 (R Foundation for Statistical Computing, Vienna, Austria). We considered *P* values less than .05 statistically significant.

RESULTS

From the INPC, we identified 2 798 709 unique vaccine recipients and 736 193 individuals with documented SARS-CoV-2 infection between November 29, 2020, and February 9, 2022. From these, we matched 267 847 vaccine recipients with the same number of infected participants (Figure 1). The demographic and clinical characteristics of the 2 groups of participants are presented in Table 1.

Infection, All-Cause Care Utilization, and Death

Cumulative incidence rates of events of interest were estimated and are presented graphically in Figure 2. Panel A shows a significantly higher cumulative incidence of infection or reinfection in vaccine recipients than those with previous infection ($P<.001$). Six months after the index date, the cumulative infection rate in the vaccinated was 6.7% (95% confidence interval [CI] = 6.6%, 6.9%), more than twice the rate in those with previous infections at 2.9% (95% CI = 2.9%, 3.0%).

Figure B (available as a supplement to the online version of this article at https://ajph.org) shows that the cumulative incidence of all-cause ED visits was significantly lower in vaccinated individuals ($P<.001$). At 6 months, 6.6% (95% CI = 6.5%, 6.7%) of the individuals with previous infection and 5.0% (95% CI = 4.9%, 5.1%) of the vaccinated individuals had recorded ED visits. Figure C (available as a supplement to the online version of this article at https://ajph.org) shows that the all-cause hospitalization rate was also significantly lower in the vaccinated ($P<.001$). Six months after the index date, 1.9% (95% CI = 1.8%, 1.9%) of the previously infected individuals and 1.2% (95% CI = 1.1%, 1.3%) of the vaccinated had recorded hospitalization. Figure D (available as a supplement to the online version of this article at https://ajph.org) shows that the mortality rate was also significantly lower in the vaccinated ($P<.001$). Six months after the index date, mortality rates were respectively 0.51% (95% CI = 0.48%, 0.54%) in the previously infected and 0.32% (95% CI = 0.29%, 0.34%) in the vaccinated.

Age-Stratified Analysis

We performed additional analyses to examine the event rates in individuals of different age groups. Results are presented in Figures B through F (available as supplements to the online version of this article at https://ajph.org). While similar patterns generally held in all age strata, the magnitudes of the estimated incidence rates varied across age groups. In children aged 19 years or younger, vaccine effectiveness against new infections was considerably less than natural immunity acquired from earlier infections (Figure B, section A).

Compared with other age groups, children had the highest incidence rates of new infections. For instance, the 6-month cumulative incidence rates of infection were, respectively, 8.1% (95% CI = 7.6%, 8.5%) and 5.2% (95% CI = 4.8%, 5.5%) for the vaccinated and previously infected. Notably, despite the higher rate of infections observed in the vaccinated children, at 6 months, the rate of all-cause ED visits in the vaccinated children was significantly lower (5.0% for the vaccinated [95% CI = 4.6%, 5.3%] vs 6.9% for the previously infected [95% CI = 6.5%, 7.3%]). The rate of all-cause hospitalization was also lower in the vaccinated (0.3% for vaccinated [95% CI = 0.3%, 0.4%] vs 0.6% for the previously infected [95% CI = 0.5%, 0.8%]; Figure C, sections B and C). Mortality rates were extremely low (< 0.1%) in both vaccinated and previously infected children; the difference was not statistically significant ($P=.5$).

In adults aged 20 to 39 years, rates of incidence infection were higher among vaccine recipients (7.8%; 95% CI = 7.6%, 8.0%) than persons with previous infections (3.2%; 95% CI = 3.0%, 3.3%) at 6 months (Figure C, section A). However, the 6-month rate of all-cause ED visit was higher in those with previous infections (7.6%; 95% CI = 7.4%, 7.8%) than in the vaccinated (5.4%; 95% CI = 5.2%, 5.6%). Similarly, the 6-month rate of hospitalization was significantly higher in the previously infected (2.1%; 95% CI = 2.0%, 2.2%) than the vaccinated (1.2%; 95% CI = 1.1%, 1.3%). The mortality rate was also higher in the previously infected (0.08%; 95% CI = 0.07%, 0.10%) than the vaccinated (0.04%; 95% CI = 0.03%, 0.07%; Figure C, sections B–D).

In adults aged 40 to 59 years, the cumulative incidence rate of infections was higher among the vaccinated (6.1%; 95% CI = 5.9%, 6.3%) than the previously infected (2.2%; 95% CI = 2.0%, 2.3%) at 6 months (Figure D, section A). However, the rate of ED visits was significantly lower in the vaccinated (4.6%; 95% CI = 4.4%, 4.8%) than the previously infected (5.4%; 95%

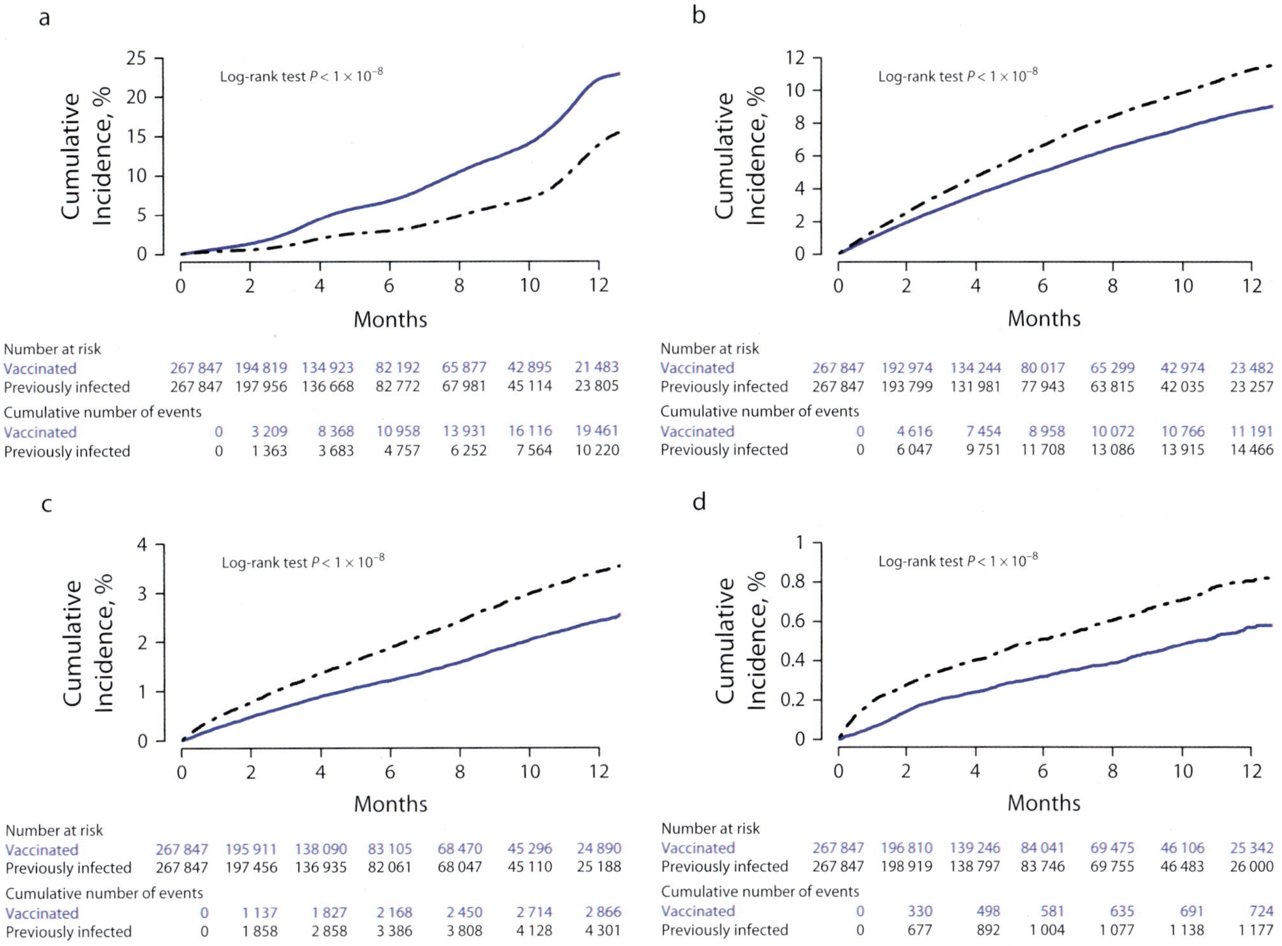

(a)

Number at risk	0	2	4	6	8	10	12
Vaccinated	267 847	194 819	134 923	82 192	65 877	42 895	21 483
Previously infected	267 847	197 956	136 668	82 772	67 981	45 114	23 805
Cumulative number of events							
Vaccinated	0	3 209	8 368	10 958	13 931	16 116	19 461
Previously infected	0	1 363	3 683	4 757	6 252	7 564	10 220

(b)

Number at risk	0	2	4	6	8	10	12
Vaccinated	267 847	192 974	134 244	80 017	65 299	42 974	23 482
Previously infected	267 847	193 799	131 981	77 943	63 815	42 035	23 257
Cumulative number of events							
Vaccinated	0	4 616	7 454	8 958	10 072	10 766	11 191
Previously infected	0	6 047	9 751	11 708	13 086	13 915	14 466

(c)

Number at risk	0	2	4	6	8	10	12
Vaccinated	267 847	195 911	138 090	83 105	68 470	45 296	24 890
Previously infected	267 847	197 456	136 935	82 061	68 047	45 110	25 188
Cumulative number of events							
Vaccinated	0	1 137	1 827	2 168	2 450	2 714	2 866
Previously infected	0	1 858	2 858	3 386	3 808	4 128	4 301

(d)

Number at risk	0	2	4	6	8	10	12
Vaccinated	267 847	196 810	139 246	84 041	69 475	46 106	25 342
Previously infected	267 847	198 919	138 797	83 746	69 755	46 483	26 000
Cumulative number of events							
Vaccinated	0	330	498	581	635	691	724
Previously infected	0	677	892	1 004	1 077	1 138	1 177

FIGURE 2— Cumulative Incidence Rates, in Vaccine Recipients and Individuals With Previous Infections, of (a) SARS-CoV-2 Infection or Reinfection, (b) Emergency Department Visit, (c) All-Cause Hospitalization, and (d) Death: SARS-COV-2 Infection, Hospitalizations, and Mortality in Vaccinated and Infected Individuals, Indiana, 2020–2022

Note. SARS-CoV-2 = severe acute respiratory syndrome coronavirus 2.

CI = 5.2%, 5.6%). All-cause hospitalization rate was also lower in the vaccinated (1.0%; 95% CI = 0.9%, 1.1%) as compared with the infected (1.4%; 95% CI = 1.3%, 1.5%). All-cause mortality rate was similarly lower in the vaccinated (0.2%; 95% CI = 0.2%, 0.3%) than in the infected (0.3%; 95% CI = 0.3%, 0.4%; Figure D, sections B–D).

In adults aged 60 to 79 years, the cumulative incidence of infections was higher in the vaccinated (3.2%; 95% CI = 2.9%, 3.5%) than the previously infected (1.9%; 95% CI = 1.7%, 2.1%) at 6 months (Figure E, section A, available as a supplement to the online version of this article at https://ajph.org). However, the rate of all-cause ED visits was lower in the vaccinated (4.6%; 95% CI = 4.3%, 4.9%) than the previously infected (5.7%; 95% CI = 5.3%, 6.0%). Rate of all-cause hospitalization was also lower in the vaccinated (2.4%; 95% CI = 2.2%, 2.6%) than in the previously infected (3.3%; 95% CI = 3.0%, 3.5%). All-cause mortality rate was similarly lower in the vaccinated (1.4%; 95% CI = 1.2%, 1.5%) than in the previously infected (2.2%; 95% CI = 2.0%, 2.4%; Figure E, sections B–D).

Finally, in adults aged 80 years or older, the vaccinated had a lower rate of hospitalization at 6 months (6.2%; 95% CI = 4.9%, 7.4%) than the previously infected (7.6%; 95% CI = 6.3%, 9.0%). All-cause mortality rate was also lower in the vaccinated (8.7%; 95% CI = 7.3%, 10.1%) than the previously infected (12.9%; 95% CI = 11.2%, 14.5%; Figure F, sections C and D).

DISCUSSION

We compared the incidence rates of SARS-CoV-2 infections, all-cause ED visits, hospitalizations, and deaths in the vaccinated and previously infected individuals living in the state of Indiana by combining medical record data and comprehensive testing and vaccination data from a statewide health information exchange and the state department of health. The analysis included 267 847 pairs of vaccine recipients and individuals with previous infections, aged between 12 and 110 years, matched on age, gender, CDC-defined COVID-19 risk scores, and dates of initial exposure (to the vaccines or the virus itself).

The study data showed that vaccination provided superior protection against all-cause ED visits, hospitalizations, and all-cause mortality compared with the levels of protection conferred by previous SARS-CoV-2 infections. Previous studies have shown that mRNA vaccines are highly effective in preventing COVID-19–related hospitalizations and mortality.[3,24,25] However, to our knowledge, no studies have directly compared the real-world protective effects of recent (i.e., 6 months) natural and vaccine-induced immunity against all-cause mortality and hospitalization in a statewide population. The study showed that while people of all age groups benefited from vaccination, reduction in mortality was especially impressive in older adults aged 60 years or older.

Interestingly, at least in the study population and at time of this analysis, natural immunity appears more effective in preventing new infections, a finding that is also reported in an earlier observational study.[26] Still, the significant reductions in all-cause health events (i.e., 24% reduction in ED visits, 37% reduction in hospitalization, and 37% reduction in mortality) in the vaccinated group are quite notable, especially considering the higher infection rate in the vaccine recipients during the same period. For states with large populations, a difference of such magnitudes could translate to hundreds or even thousands of lives saved.

Compared with COVID-19–specific outcomes, all-cause hospitalization and mortality rates used in the current analysis may be more informative on the health consequences of SARS-CoV-2 infection and protective effects of vaccination.[27] As the study indicates, the strong natural immunity acquired from a previous infection does not appear to fully compensate for the detrimental effects of the initial infection. Therefore, our findings reinforce the importance of vaccination as an essential public health measure to counter the health impacts of the SARS-CoV-2 pandemic. The significantly higher all-cause mortality observed in individuals with previous infection suggested that reliance on natural immunity to avoid negative SARS-CoV-2 health consequences is not a prudent strategy given the safe and readily available vaccines.

In this research, we have employed a matched cohort study design, an approach used by other large population-based vaccine-effectiveness studies.[3] Compared with alternative methods, such as the test-negative design,[28] matched cohorts directly emulate the structure of a clinical trial. Although the design provides no guarantee of a causal interpretation, estimation and inference are straightforward.[29] The convenience of the analysis, however, comes at the expense of matching costs: among other things, many vaccinated and infected individuals were excluded from the analysis for lack of an appropriate match. We carefully selected the matching variables to minimize biases associated with excluding otherwise eligible participants. For the index date, we opted to use the date of the initial SARS-CoV-2 exposure plus 30 days to accommodate the temporal uncertainty in immunity development: previous studies showed that full immunity was conveyed by the vaccines 7 to 14 days after the second dose,[30] whereas robust humoral and cellular immune response occur 5 to 15 days following the onset of symptoms, and antibodies peak within the first few weeks.[13,31,32]

Well-matched cohorts, however, do not preclude the possibility of remnant differences between the comparison groups, especially in characteristics not captured by the matching variables. For example, in the present context, one might suspect that the lower mortality among the vaccine recipients was attributable to their tendency for risk-averse behaviors, such as mask-wearing, hand sanitizing, and social distancing.[33] But such an interpretation was not supported by the data showing a higher incidence of infection among vaccine recipients. In addition, the outcome of primary interest, all-cause mortality, is an objective metric that can be readily captured in both vaccinated and previously infected groups with equal accuracy. As a result, we contend that, despite the study's observational nature, the comprehensive real-world data source, the large sample size, the temporally matched participant characteristics, and the consistent findings across different age groups lend credibility to the investigation.

While the findings related to the ED visits, hospital admissions, and deaths align with previous research,[4,5,18,34] few real-world population-based studies have compared the effectiveness of protection against SARS-CoV-2 for natural infections and vaccinations.[35,36]

Although our results suggest that natural immunity provides greater protection against subsequent infections than vaccines, residual confounding attributable to health-seeking behavior may still have an impact on these results.[37] If the rate of symptomatic testing for SARS-CoV-2 infection is greater among vaccinated individuals (a quantity unmeasured in our study), vaccine effectiveness would be underestimated.

The matched cohort design, while effective for comparing the relative proactive effects of natural and vaccine-induced immunity, presents significant challenges for examining the effects of different vaccines or vaccine doses, as well as their response to specific variants of SARS-CoV-2. In this research, we did not examine the differences among vaccine types, doses, and viral variants, which had distinct temporal patterns in the pandemic, to avoid an over-complication of the matching process. Notwithstanding this limitation, we showed that the all-cause mortality rate was 37% lower in vaccine recipients compared with individuals with previous infections 6 months after the index date. The reductions in ED visits and hospital admissions were respectively 24% and 37%. The findings highlight the real-world benefits of vaccination and allude to the health consequences of SARS-CoV-2 after the initial exposure. AJPH

ABOUT THE AUTHORS

Wanzhu Tu and Pengyue Zhang are with the Indiana University School of Medicine and the Fairbanks School of Public Health, Indianapolis. Peter Embi and Shaun Grannis are with the Indiana University School of Medicine, Indianapolis. Anna Roberts, Katie S. Allen, and Jennifer Williams are with the Regenstrief Institute Inc, Indianapolis.

CORRESPONDENCE

Correspondence should be sent to Shaun Grannis, Regenstrief Institute Inc, 1101 W 10th St, Indianapolis, IN 46202 (e-mail: sgrannis@regenstrief.org). Reprints can be ordered at https://ajph.org by clicking the "Reprints" link.

PUBLICATION INFORMATION

Full Citation: Tu W, Zhang P, Roberts A, et al. SARS-CoV-2 infection, hospitalization, and death in vaccinated and infected individuals by age groups in Indiana, 2021–2022. *Am J Public Health*. 2023; 113(1):96–104.

Acceptance Date: September 1, 2022.

DOI: https://doi.org/10.2105/AJPH.2022.307112

CONTRIBUTORS

W. Tu, P. Zhang, P. Embi, and S. Grannis conceptualized and designed this study. W. Tu, P. Zhang, A. Roberts, P. Embi, and S. Grannis were responsible for acquisition, analysis, or interpretation of data. Primary writing for this article was completed by W. Tu with critical revision by P. Embi, S. Grannis, and P. Zhang. All statistical analysis was completed by P. Zhang and W. Tu. Administrative, technical, and material support was provided by K. S. Allen and J. Williams.

ACKNOWLEDGMENTS

We would like to thank the Regenstrief Institute Inc for their support of faculty and staff effort.

CONFLICTS OF INTEREST

The authors have no conflicts of interest related to this study.

HUMAN PARTICIPANT PROTECTION

This study was reviewed and approved as exempt by the Indiana University institutional review board before data collection and analysis.

REFERENCES

1. Bajema KL, Dahl RM, Prill MM, et al. Effectiveness of COVID-19 mRNA vaccines against COVID-19-associated hospitalization—five Veterans Affairs medical centers, United States, February 1–August 6, 2021. *MMWR Morb Mortal Wkly Rep*. 2021;70(37):1294–1299. https://doi.org/10.15585/mmwr.mm7037e3
2. Livingston EH, Malani PN, Creech CB. The Johnson & Johnson Vaccine for COVID-19. *JAMA*. 2021;325(15):1575. https://doi.org/10.1001/jama.2021.2927
3. Dagan N, Barda N, Kepten E, et al. BNT162b2 mRNA Covid-19 vaccine in a nationwide mass vaccination setting. *N Engl J Med*. 2021;384(15):1412–1423. https://doi.org/10.1056/NEJMoa2101765
4. Thompson MG, Stenehjem E, Grannis S, et al. Effectiveness of Covid-19 vaccines in ambulatory and inpatient care wettings. *N Engl J Med*. 2021; 385(15):1355–1371. https://doi.org/10.1056/NEJMoa2110362
5. Grannis SJ, Rowley EA, Ong TC, et al. Interim estimates of COVID-19 vaccine effectiveness against COVID-19-associated emergency department or urgent care clinic encounters and hospitalizations among adults during SARS-CoV-2 B.1.617.2 (Delta) variant predominance—nine states, June–August 2021. *MMWR Morb Mortal Wkly Rep*. 2021;70(37):1291–1293. https://doi.org/10.15585/mmwr.mm7037e2
6. Natarajan K, Prasad N, Dascomb K, et al. Effectiveness of homologous and heterologous COVID-19 booster doses following 1 Ad.26.COV2.S (Janssen [Johnson & Johnson]) vaccine dose against COVID-19–associated emergency department and urgent care encounters and hospitalizations among adults—VISION Network, 10 states, December 2021–March 2022. *MMWR Morb Mortal Wkly Rep*. 2022;71(13):495–502. https://doi.org/10.15585/mmwr.mm7113e2
7. Lipsitch M, Krammer F, Regev-Yochay G, Lustig Y, Balicer RD. SARS-CoV-2 breakthrough infections in vaccinated individuals: measurement, causes and impact. *Nat Rev Immunol*. 2022;22(1):57–65. https://doi.org/10.1038/s41577-021-00662-4
8. Ferdinands JM, Rao S, Dixon BE, et al. Waning 2-dose and 3-dose effectiveness of mRNA vaccines against COVID-19-associated emergency department and urgent care encounters and hospitalizations among adults during periods of delta and omicron variant predominance—VISION Network, 10 states, August 2021–January 2022. *MMWR Morb Mortal Wkly Rep*. 2022;71(7):255–263. https://doi.org/10.15585/mmwr.mm7107e2
9. Scott J, Richterman A, Cevik M. COVID-19 vaccination: evidence of waning immunity is overstated. *BMJ*. 2021;374(2320):n2320. https://doi.org/10.1136/bmj.n2320
10. Tregoning JS, Flight KE, Higham SL, Wang Z, Pierce BF. Progress of the COVID-19 vaccine effort: viruses, vaccines and variants versus efficacy, effectiveness and escape. *Nat Rev Immunol*. 2021;21(10):626–636. https://doi.org/10.1038/s41577-021-00592-1
11. Goldberg Y, Mandel M, Bar-On YM, et al. Waning immunity after the BNT162b2 vaccine in Israel. *N Engl J Med*. 2021;385(24):e85. https://doi.org/10.1056/NEJMoa2114228
12. Thomas SJ, Moreira ED Jr, Kitchin N, et al. Safety and efficacy of the BNT162b2 mRNA COVID-19 vaccine through 6 months. *N Engl J Med*. 2021; 385(19):1761–1773. https://doi.org/10.1056/NEJMoa2110345
13. Post N, Eddy D, Huntley C, et al. Antibody response to SARS-CoV-2 infection in humans: a systematic review. *PLoS One*. 2020;15(12):e0244126. https://doi.org/10.1371/journal.pone.0244126
14. Shrotri M, van Schalkwyk MCI, Post N, et al. T cell response to SARS-CoV-2 infection in humans: a systematic review. *PLoS One*. 2021;16(1):e0245532. https://doi.org/10.1371/journal.pone.0245532
15. Hall VJ, Foulkes S, Charlett A, et al. SARS-CoV-2 infection rates of antibody-positive compared with antibody-negative health-care workers in England: a large, multicentre, prospective cohort study (SIREN). *Lancet*. 2021;397(10283):1459–1469. https://doi.org/10.1016/S0140-6736(21)00675-9
16. Hansen CH, Michlmayr D, Gubbels SM, Molbak K, Ethelberg S. Assessment of protection against reinfection with SARS-CoV-2 among 4 million PCR-tested individuals in Denmark in 2020: a population-level observational study. *Lancet*.

2021;397(10280):1204–1212. https://doi.org/10.1016/S0140-6736(21)00575-4

17. Vitale J, Mumoli N, Clerici P, et al. Assessment of SARS-CoV-2 reinfection 1 year after primary infection in a population in Lombardy, Italy. *JAMA Intern Med.* 2021;181(10):1407–1408. https://doi.org/10.1001/jamainternmed.2021.2959
18. Bozio CH, Grannis SJ, Naleway AL, et al. Laboratory-confirmed COVID-19 among adults hospitalized with COVID-19-like illness with infection-induced or mRNA vaccine-induced SARS-CoV-2 immunity—nine states, January–September 2021. *MMWR Morb Mortal Wkly Rep.* 2021;70(44):1539–1544. https://doi.org/10.15585/mmwr.mm7044e1
19. León TM, Dorabawila V, Nelson L, et al. COVID-19 cases and hospitalizations by COVID-19 vaccination status and previous COVID-19 diagnosis—California and New York, May–November 2021. *MMWR Morb Mortal Wkly Rep.* 2022;71(4):125–131. https://doi.org/10.15585/mmwr.mm7104e1
20. Shenai MB, Rahme R, Noorchashm H. Equivalency of protection from natural immunity in COVID-19 recovered versus fully vaccinated persons: a systematic review and pooled analysis. *Cureus.* 2021;13(10):e19102. https://doi.org/10.7759/cureus.19102
21. Overhage JM. The Indiana health information exchange. In: Dixon BE, ed. *Health Information Exchange: Navigating and Managing a Network of Health Information Systems.* Elsevier; 2016;1:267–279.
22. Dixon BE, Grannis SJ, McAndrews C, et al. Leveraging data visualization and a statewide health information exchange to support COVID-19 surveillance and response: application of public health informatics. *J Am Med Inform Assoc.* 2021;28(7):1363–1373. https://doi.org/10.1093/jamia/ocab004
23. Grannis SJ, Overhage JM, McDonald CJ. Analysis of identifier performance using a deterministic linkage algorithm. *Proc AMIA Symp.* 2002:305–309.
24. Tenforde MW, Patel MM, Ginde AA, et al. Effectiveness of SARS-CoV-2 mRNA vaccines for preventing COVID-19 hospitalizations in the United States. *Clin Infect Dis.* 2022;74(9):1515–1524. https://doi.org/10.1101/2021.07.08.21259776
25. Xu S, Huang R, Sy LS, et al. COVID-19 vaccination and non–COVID-19 mortality risk—seven integrated health care organizations, United States, December 14, 2020–July 31, 2021. *MMWR Morb Mortal Wkly Rep.* 2021;70(43):1520–1524. https://doi.org/10.15585/mmwr.mm7043e2
26. Gazit S, Shlezinger R, Perez G, et al. Severe acute respiratory syndrome coronavirus 2 (SARS-CoV-2) naturally acquired immunity vs. vaccine-induced immunity, reinfections versus breakthrough infections: a retrospective cohort study. *Clin Infect Dis.* 2022;75(1):e545–e551 https://doi.org/10.1093/cid/ciac262
27. Wanga V, Chevinsky JR, Dimitrov LV, et al. Long-term symptoms among adults tested for SARS-CoV-2—United States, January 2020–April 2021. *MMWR Morb Mortal Wkly Rep.* 2021;70(36):1235–1241. https://doi.org/10.15585/mmwr.mm7036a1
28. Sullivan SG, Tchetgen Tchetgen EJ, Cowling BJ. Theoretical basis of the test-negative study design for assessment of influenza vaccine effectiveness. *Am J Epidemiol.* 2016;184(5):345–353. https://doi.org/10.1093/aje/kww064
29. Hernán MA, Robins JM. Using big data to emulate a target trial when a randomized trial is not available. *Am J Epidemiol.* 2016;183(8):758–764. https://doi.org/10.1093/aje/kwv254
30. Polack FP, Thomas SJ, Kitchin N, et al. Safety and efficacy of the BNT162b2 mRNA COVID-19 vaccine. *N Engl J Med.* 2020;383(27):2603–2615. https://doi.org/10.1056/NEJMoa2034577
31. Röltgen K, Powell AE, Wirz OF, et al. Defining the features and duration of antibody responses to SARS-CoV-2 infection associated with disease severity and outcome. *Sci Immunol.* 2020;5(54):eabe0240. https://doi.org/10.1126/sciimmunol.abe0240
32. Gudbjartsson DF, Norddahl GL, Melsted P, et al. Humoral immune response to SARS-CoV-2 in Iceland. *N Engl J Med.* 2020;383(18):1724–1734. https://doi.org/10.1056/NEJMoa2026116
33. Petherick A, Goldszmidt R, Andrade EB, et al. A worldwide assessment of changes in adherence to COVID-19 protective behaviours and hypothesized pandemic fatigue. *Nat Hum Behav.* 2021;5(9):1145–1160. https://doi.org/10.1038/s41562-021-01181-x
34. Johnson AG, Amin AB, Ali AR, et al. COVID-19 incidence and death rates among unvaccinated and fully vaccinated adults with and without booster doses during periods of delta and omicron variant emergence—25 US jurisdictions, April 4–December 25, 2021. *MMWR Morb Mortal Wkly Rep.* 2022;71(4):132–138. https://doi.org/10.15585/mmwr.mm7104e2
35. Elliott P, Haw D, Wang H, et al. Exponential growth, high prevalence of SARS-CoV-2, and vaccine effectiveness associated with the Delta variant. *Science.* 2021;374(6574):eabl9551. https://doi.org/10.1126/science.abl9551
36. Hall V, Foulkes S, Insalata F, et al. Protection against SARS-CoV-2 after COVID-19 vaccination and previous infection. *N Engl J Med.* 2022;386(13):1207–1220. https://doi.org/10.1056/NEJMoa2118691
37. Jackson ML, Nelson JC. The test-negative design for estimating influenza vaccine effectiveness. *Vaccine.* 2013;31(17):2165–2168. https://doi.org/10.1016/j.vaccine.2013.02.053

A Community Health Worker–Based Intervention on Anthropometric Outcomes of Children Aged 3 to 21 Months in Urban Pakistan, 2019–2021

Abu S. Shonchoy, PhD, Agha A. Akram, PhD, Mahrukh Khan, BSc, Hina Khalid, PhD, Sidra Mazhar, MSc, Akib Khan, MS, and Takashi Kurosaki, PhD

Objectives. To evaluate the impact of a community health worker–based "in-home growth monitoring with counseling" (IHGMC) intervention on anthropometric outcomes in Pakistan, where 38% of children younger than 5 years are stunted.

Methods. We used an individual, single-blind, step-wedge randomized controlled trial and a pure control group recruited at endline. We based the analysis on an intention-to-treat estimation using the coarsened exact matching (CEM) method for sample selection among treatments and the control. We conducted the baseline in July 2019 and completed endline in September–October 2021. We recruited 1639 households (treated: 1188; control: 451) with children aged 3 to 21 months who were residing in an urban informal settlement area. The CEM sample used for analysis numbered 1046 (treated: 636; control: 410). The intervention continued for 6 months.

Results. Compared with the control group, the height-for-age *z*-score in the IHGMC group increased by 0.58 SD (95% confidence interval [CI] = 0.33, 0.83; $P = .001$) and the weight-for-age *z*-score by 0.43 SD (95% CI = 0.20, 0.67; $P < .01$), measured at endline.

Conclusions. IHGMC substantially improved child anthropometric outcomes in disadvantaged localities, and this impact persisted during the COVID-19 pandemic.

Trial Registration. AER-RCT registry (AEARCTR-0003248). (*Am J Public Health*. 2023;113(1):105–114. https://doi.org/10.2105/AJPH.2022.307111)

AJPH January 2023, Vol 113, No. 1

Globally, 1 in 4 children younger than 5 years suffers from linear growth faltering,[1] with the highest prevalence in South Asia and sub-Saharan Africa.[2] Stunting (low height-for-age *z*-score [HAZ] < -2) remains a critical public health challenge as it reduces lifetime earnings, hinders cognitive development, and leads to high mortality rates.[3] The COVID-19 pandemic has raised concerns about reversals to improvements in childhood nutrition.[4] These concerns have been met with a renewed emphasis on the importance of mobilizing resources for nutrition[5] and an urgency to increase resilience to malnutrition during times of crises,[6] such as a pandemic.

Research suggests that primary caregivers play a key role in child development.[7] Caregivers are the first point of contact for children, and their engagement is crucial to ensure adequate physical, cognitive, social, and emotional development. Consequently, community health worker (CHW) programs, globally[8] and in Pakistan,[9] leverage regular contact with primary caregivers to improve child health outcomes. Existing CHW-based public health delivery programs, which have shown promise in maternal and child health[10] by encouraging health-care-facility utilization by caregivers, have produced modest gains in child health (typically lower than a 0.25 SD gain in HAZ).[11–13]

Several limitations remain, as these programs predominantly focus on resource and knowledge constraints but provide little attention to behavioral interventions such as engaging caregivers with continuous feedback on the growth measures of their children.[14,15] Programs that use cash transfers to address resource constraints show limited impact.[16] Physical growth promotion programs mostly operate through facility-based growth monitoring[17] and rarely focus on regular home-based growth surveillance by CHWs, with the exception of a handful of small sample studies.[12,18] Programs that simply integrate growth charts into the community-based interventions—without regular growth monitoring—do not see any impact because caregivers often fail to comprehend growth trajectories.[19] The complementarity of regular growth monitoring and counseling for caregivers is essential, as it improves the understanding of child care inputs and physical development, particularly in marginalized communities.

The few studies that explored behavioral interventions have shown limited effect on child growth. One of the first rigorous studies on regular growth monitoring with a growth chart, the South Indian Trial,[18] did not find any additional benefit from growth monitoring. The study setting was small (12 villages in Tamil Nadu), focused on weight measures, and was executed by 1 selected mother in the village. Its impact measures also did not isolate the impact of growth monitoring from that of the growth chart. A related study, conducted in Zambia,[20] focused on home-based growth monitoring (life-sized posters installed in homes to demonstrate children's age-appropriate height) and community-based growth monitoring along with nutritional supplements. This study found modest positive effects on growth among previously malnourished children; however, the study suffered from a lack of professionally measured anthropometrics at regular intervals and did not assess complementarities between monitoring and counseling. Thus far, the existing literature is inconclusive and lacks sufficient evidence in evaluating the impact of regular in-home anthropometric monitoring and counseling executed by trained CHWs.

Motivated by this concern, we tested in-home growth monitoring coupled with nutrition counseling in Pakistan, a lower-middle-income country in South Asia with high levels of childhood stunting: 38% of all children younger than 5 years are stunted, although this figure is lower in urban areas (31%) and for children aged 6 to 8 months (18%).[21] We chose to study the intervention in an informal urban settlement, a setting that hosts marginalized populations but rarely receives health or nutritional aid. Additionally, our study was conducted during a global pandemic, which—as many experts fear—threatens child nutritional development, especially in areas where health facilities are being closed or partially functional.[22]

METHODS

Our main sample for the impact analysis came from a randomized controlled trial, which we conducted in Gulshan-e-Sikandarabad, an urban informal settlement located in Karachi, Pakistan. Households with at least 1 child aged 3 to 21 months were eligible for this trial. An independent survey team listed 4166 households, found 1823 of them to be eligible for our trial, and administered a baseline survey (July 2019) to the biological mother and caregiver of the child, capturing demographics, socioeconomics, and child anthropometrics. If more than 1 eligible child was present in the household, the youngest one was chosen. This process continued until 1188 eligible households completed the baseline survey and were randomly allocated to 1 of 3 treatment arms (1:1:1) entailing 396 households in each group, as follows: T1: monthly in-home growth monitoring with counseling (IHGMC); T2: IHGMC with a poster-sized HAZ-based growth monitoring interactive chart; T3: IHGMC plus growth charts (as in T2) complemented with a monthly unconditional cash transfer (fixed amount of Rs 400 [$11.91 in purchasing power parity]), with a suggestion to use the amount for children's food. This intervention continued for 6 months (September 2019–February 2020) and ended just before the COVID-19 outbreak. The balance table on treatment assignment is reported in Table A10 of Appendix A (available as a supplement to the online version of this article at http://www.ajph.org).

An endline survey was administered 13 months after the start of intervention activities (September–October 2020), with a no-contact period of 7 months. The endline survey was timed this way to allow better understanding of the persistence of gains in child health, especially as measured during the pandemic. At this time, we added a pure control group by surveying an additional 451 households, recruited from the subset of eligible households in the original list of 4166 households generated during our initial community census, utilizing the same eligibility criteria of having a child aged 3 to 21 months and presence of the household in the community at the time of baseline. Adding this pure control group allowed us to compare the treatment impact with a no-intervention scenario, going beyond the ambit of the original randomized controlled trial (a detailed timeline is given in online Appendix B).

AJPH January 2023, Vol 113, No. 1

Randomization, Matching, and Masking

We initially designed a sample size of 400 households per intervention group to detect an effect size of 0.3 SD in HAZ between any of the 3 treatment arms, with a power of 0.8 and an α level of 0.05, unconditional on covariates. This statistical power remained similar when we used a matched sample.

We used coarsened exact matching (CEM) to select our sample for analysis from the treatment and control groups, since we added the control group to an ongoing randomized controlled trial. We used CEM to match on household size, child's age at baseline, father's education, mother's education, and language.[23] We improved the matching by reducing the L1 distance (an objective measure of how different the raw, unmatched control and treatment samples are from each other) from 0.94 to 0.57. Details of CEM are provided in online Appendix D, and the balance on observables for the matched sample are shown in Table A11 of online Appendix A.

The nature of our intervention did not allow full masking of participants to the CHWs. Although the team of investigators was masked, the data collection team was not strictly blinded to intervention group assignment since the endline survey asked about some of the treatment-related activities, which allowed them to predict individual treatment allocation (online Appendix E). The detailed procedures on team recruitment and training and on intervention operational protocols are given in online Appendixes H, G, and E, respectively.

Outcomes

The primary outcome measures were HAZ, where height was measured using infantometers and stadiometers, and weight-for-age *z*-score (WAZ), where weight was measured using weighing scales (for detailed procedures, see online Appendix G). We calculated HAZ scores using the in-built Stata package "zscore06" (StataCorp LP, College Station, TX) in accordance with the World Health Organization (WHO) Child Growth Standards for children younger than 5 years. Our secondary outcomes were binary indicators for stunted and severely stunted (i.e., 2 SD and 3 SD below the median HAZ score of the reference population, respectively, underlying the WHO Child Growth Standards) as well as binary indicators for underweight and severe underweight (i.e., 2 SD and 3 SD, respectively, below the median WAZ score from the WHO Child Growth Standards).[24] Another secondary outcome was weight-for-height *z*-score (WHZ), which captured the weight of the child compared with their height as well as 2 binary variables: wasting (i.e., WHZ < -2 SD) and severely wasted (i.e., WHZ < -3 SD). We measured height and weight in duplicates, following the WHO Multicenter Growth Reference Study method.[25] Additional variables analyzed were caregiver knowledge, quality of diet, and the home environment (online Appendix F).

Statistical Analysis

All our analyses followed an intention-to-treat (ITT) estimation on the matched sample. CEM yielded a total sample of 1046 households across the control and treatments (198 in T1, 208 in T2, 230 in T3, and 410 in the control), with a matching control:T1:T2:T3 ratio of 1:0.48:0.51:0.56. Our ITT estimation generated causal effects of treatment on outcome variables. ITT estimates minimize bias through selective take-up of the intervention, providing lower bound impact estimates. We employed ITT regression analysis using binary variables to designate treatment status (versions with individual- and household-level covariates are reported in Tables A15 through A23 of online Appendix A) to evaluate the impact of the 3 treatments, using Stata 14 with Huber–White robust standard errors. We used the same strategy for the treatment component–specific analysis (termed "reclassification"), where we estimated the ITT impacts using binary indicators for treatment components: counseling = T1+T2+T3 (n = 636); growth chart = T2+T3 (n = 438); and cash transfer = T3 (n = 230). We present ITT coefficient estimates (means) with 95% confidence intervals (CIs) and *P* values using outcomes measured at endline. We estimated heterogeneous treatment effects by interacting treatment status with child's gender, marginalized ethnicity dummy, and age at baseline (online Appendix C). Additionally, we used propensity score matching as a robustness check for our estimates.

RESULTS

Of the 4166 households assessed for eligibility at baseline, 1823 were found eligible, of which 1188 were employed for the intervention (online Figure A7). Of these, 5 households witnessed a death or injury of the child (< 1%) and 202 households (17%) could not be recontacted for program implementation through a combination of weak address systems (typical of informal urban settlements) and migration out of the neighborhood. Thus, our program implementation sample was 981 households (83% of baseline sample). Of these, we successfully reinterviewed 790 households at endline (81% of implementation sample); 58 households refused to be reinterviewed (5%), 11 exceeded our interview rescheduling threshold of 3 attempts (1%), 9 were located but were absent despite multiple attempts (1%), and 113 had moved out of the community (10%).

Our total available endline sample was 1241 households: 790 households from the original randomized controlled trial sample and 451 recruited to serve as the control. After we matched using CEM, our final analysis sample was 1046 households. The characteristics of these 2 groups were similar: the control arm children were 55% male and 45% female whereas the corresponding numbers in the treatment arms were 52% male and 48% female. Mother's literacy rate in this community was low: 68% of mothers had not attended at least 1 year of schooling across the control and treatment samples. Households in treatment and control were balanced across all 5 neighborhood categories. In terms of ethnicity, the proportion of historically marginalized groups was balanced across the control and treatments at 25% and 24%, respectively. Detailed descriptive statistics for the study sample are given in Table 1.

Our first set of results compared the matched control with any treatment

TABLE 1— Demographic Characteristics of the Matched Sample: Pakistan, September–October 2021

	Control Group, Mean ±SD or No. (%)	Treatment Group, Mean ±SD or No. (%)			
		T1	T2	T3	All Treatments
Household size, no.	7.84 ±4.32	8.73 ±4.44	9.09 ±4.55	8.50 ±4.15	8.77 ±4.38
Child's age, y	25.70 ±6.80	26.11 ±5.73	25.48 ±5.68	25.53 ±5.81	25.69 ±5.74
Father's education					
Not literate[a]	223 (54.52)	91 (46.19)	104 (50.24)	101 (44.10)	296 (46.76)
Literate	186 (45.48)	106 (53.81)	103 (49.76)	128 (55.90)	337 (53.24)
Mother's education					
Not literate[a]	278 (67.80)	135 (68.18)	144 (69.23)	152 (66.09)	431 (67.77)
Literate	132 (32.20)	63 (31.82)	64 (30.77)	78 (33.91)	205 (32.23)
Neighborhood					
Neighborhood 1	158 (38.73)	70 (35.35)	77 (37.02)	73 (31.74)	220 (34.59)
Neighborhood 2	66 (16.18)	31 (15.66)	42 (20.19)	55 (23.91)	128 (20.13)
Neighborhood 3	32 (7.84)	25 (12.63)	19 (9.14)	23 (10.00)	67 (10.53)
Neighborhood 4	77 (18.87)	36 (18.18)	40 (19.23)	43 (18.70)	119 (18.71)
Neighborhood 5	75 (18.38)	36 (18.18)	30 (14.42)	36 (15.65)	102 (16.04)
Language					
Urdu	3 (0.73)	2 (1.01)	2 (0.96)	2 (0.87)	6 (0.94)
Sindhi	6 (1.46)	3 (1.52)	2 (0.96)	1 (0.44)	6 (0.94)
Punjabi	56 (13.66)	16 (8.08)	19 (9.14)	18 (7.83)	53 (8.33)
Pashto	278 (67.80)	146 (73.74)	166 (79.81)	179 (77.83)	491 (77.20)
Saraiki	64 (15.61)	30 (15.15)	19 (9.14)	29 (12.61)	78 (12.26)
Other	3 (0.73)	1 (0.51)	0 (0.0)	1 (0.44)	2 (0.31)
Child's gender					
Female	184 (44.88)	104 (52.53)	87 (41.83)	112 (48.70)	303 (47.64)
Male	226 (55.12)	94 (47.47)	121 (58.17)	118 (51.30)	333 (52.36)
Marginalized ethnicity					
Other	307 (74.88)	146 (73.74)	162 (77.88)	170 (73.91)	478 (75.16)
Marginalized	103 (25.12)	52 (26.26)	46 (22.12)	60 (26.09)	158 (24.84)
Total sample	410	198	208	230	636

Note. T1 = monthly in-home growth monitoring with counseling (IHGMC); T2 = IHGMC with a poster-sized HAZ (height-for-age *z*-score)–based growth monitoring interactive chart; T3 = IHGMC plus growth charts (as in T2) complemented with a monthly unconditional cash transfer.

[a]"Not Literate" is a category for no schooling or incomplete schooling: the parent had not completed at least 1 year of schooling (i.e., was illiterate) or had not completed grade 1 or attended vocational training or madrasa education.

to quantify the impact of treatment at the time of the COVID-19 pandemic (Figure 1). Aggregate treatment estimates showed an increase in HAZ by 0.42 SD (95% CI = 0.23, 0.61; $P < .001$) compared with the control mean of −1.86 SD. The prevalence of stunting was reduced by 10 percentage points (95% CI = −0.17, −0.03; $P < .001$), and the prevalence of severe stunting was reduced by 5 percentage points (95% CI = −0.10, 0.00; $P = .04$) in the treated group compared with the control. We also found improvements in weight-related measures: a 0.25 SD increase in WAZ (95% CI = 0.07, 0.44; $P = .01$), a 6-percentage-point reduction in cases of underweight (95% CI = −0.12, 0.01; $P = .07$), and a 5-percentage-point reduction in cases of severely underweight (95% CI = −0.10, −0.01; $P = .02$). These estimates are robust to alternative matching (i.e., propensity score matching as reported in Table A14 of online Appendix A).

Next, as shown in Figure 2, we observed that T1 showed the largest improvements, with a statistically significant gain in HAZ of 0.58 SD (95% CI = 0.33, 0.83; $P < .001$), and reductions in stunting (−10 percentage points; 95% CI = −0.19, −0.01; $P = .02$) and severe stunting (−7 percentage points; 95% CI = −0.13, −0.01; $P = .03$). We also saw gains in WAZ (0.43 SD; 95% CI = 0.20, 0.67; $P < .001$), and reductions in underweight (−9 percentage points; 95% CI = −0.16, −0.01; $P = .03$) and severely underweight (−7 percentage points; 95% CI = −0.12, −0.02; $P = .01$). Compared with the control, T2 and T3 also largely followed the same direction as T1, although the magnitude of gains in HAZ and WAZ, and the reductions in stunting, severe stunting, underweight, and severe underweight, were not as large as in T1. None of our treatments had a statistically discernible impact at the conventional level on WHZ, wasted, and severely wasted compared with the control. Furthermore, as shown in Figure A1 and Table A3 of online Appendix A, reclassified treatment component–specific estimates demonstrate similar conclusions as estimated before.

Next, we estimated 2-way interactions (Figure 3) to understand if the

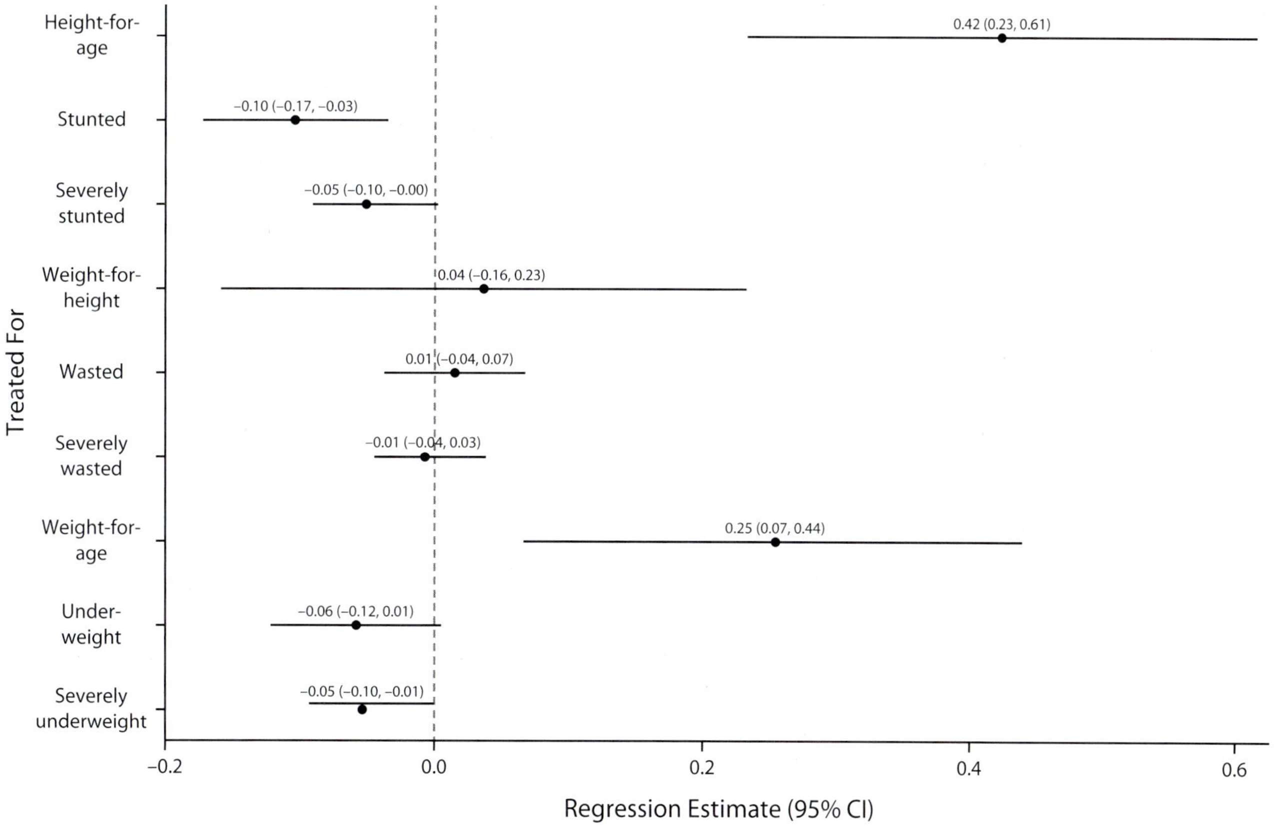

FIGURE 1— Aggregated Treatment Effect of Intervention on Primary and Secondary Outcomes: Pakistan, September–October 2021

Note. CI=confidence interval; T1 = monthly in-home growth monitoring with counseling (IHGMC); T2 = IHGMC with a poster-sized HAZ (height-for-age *z*-score)–based growth monitoring interactive chart; T3 = IHGMC plus growth charts (as in T2) complemented with a monthly unconditional cash transfer.

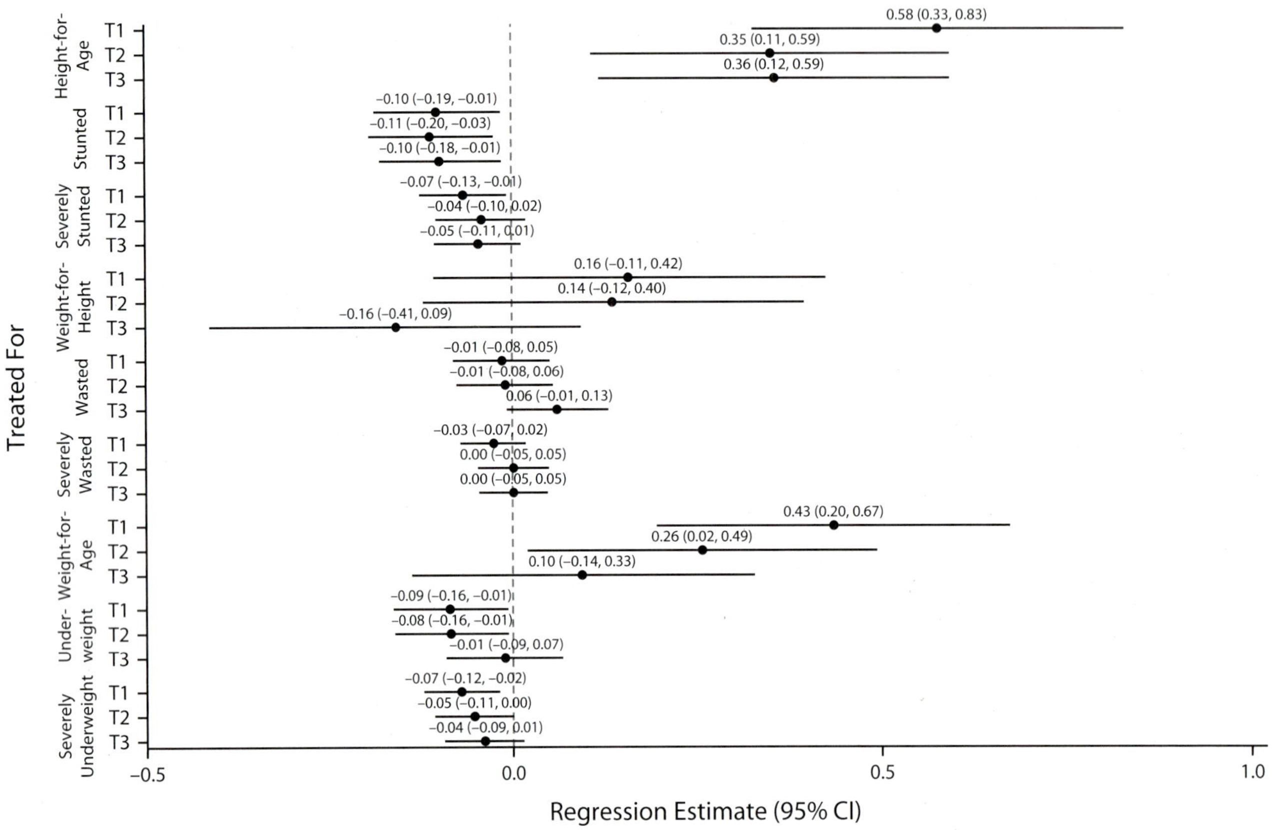

FIGURE 2— Disaggregated Treatment Effect of Intervention on Primary and Secondary Outcomes: Pakistan, September–October 2021

Note. CI = confidence interval; T1 = monthly in-home growth monitoring with counseling (IHGMC); T2 = IHGMC with a poster-sized HAZ (height-for-age *z*-score)–based growth monitoring interactive chart; T3 = IHGMC plus growth charts (as in T2) complemented with a monthly unconditional cash transfer.

effect of the treatments was different among girls and boys. The results showed that relative to girls, boys in T3 tended to have a higher HAZ (0.46 SD; 95% CI = −0.01, 0.94; $P = .05$) with an associated reduction in severe stunting (−13 percentage points; 95% CI = −0.25, −0.02; $P = .03$). Additionally, male children in T3 saw increased WAZ (0.63 SD; 95% CI = 0.17, 1.09; $P = .01$), and reduced cases of being underweight (−14 percentage points; 95% CI = −0.30, 0.02; $P = .08$) and severely underweight (−19 percentage points; 95% CI = −0.29, −0.08; $P < .001$). Finally, boys in T3 also saw increased WHZ (0.60 SD; 95% CI = 0.10, 1.11; $P = .02$) and a reduction in cases of severe wasting (−14 percentage points; 95% CI = −0.23, −0.04; $P < .001$). We found broadly similar results in reclassified treatment component estimates (Figure A2 and Table A5 of online Appendix A): male children in households that received a cash transfer had higher WAZ (0.61 SD; 95% CI = 0.12, 1.09; $P = .01$) along with a lower probability of being severely underweight (−16 percentage points; 95% CI = −0.26, −0.05; $P < .001$), and higher WHZ (0.61 SD; 95% CI = 0.04, 1.19; $P = .04$) along with a lower probability of being severely wasted (−13 percentage points; 95% CI = −0.23, −0.03; $P = .01$). We did not see a statistically significant increase in HAZ and related decreases in the probability of stunting. The other program components (IHGMC and growth chart) did not suggest any statistically significant difference by gender. Heterogeneity effects by child age and caste were inconclusive (Figures A3–A6 and Tables A6–A9 of online Appendix A).

Finally, we investigated the measures of caregiver knowledge, quality of diet, and the home environment that might have contributed to our findings (Table B2 of online Appendix B). There were 2 results of note. First, we found that children in T1 were given a 0.09 SD (95% CI = 0.01, 0.18; $P = .04$) larger quantity of dairy products compared with the control, measured as a standardized difference of an index for consuming multiple dairy food (index creation process detailed in online Appendix F). Second, we found that caregivers in T2

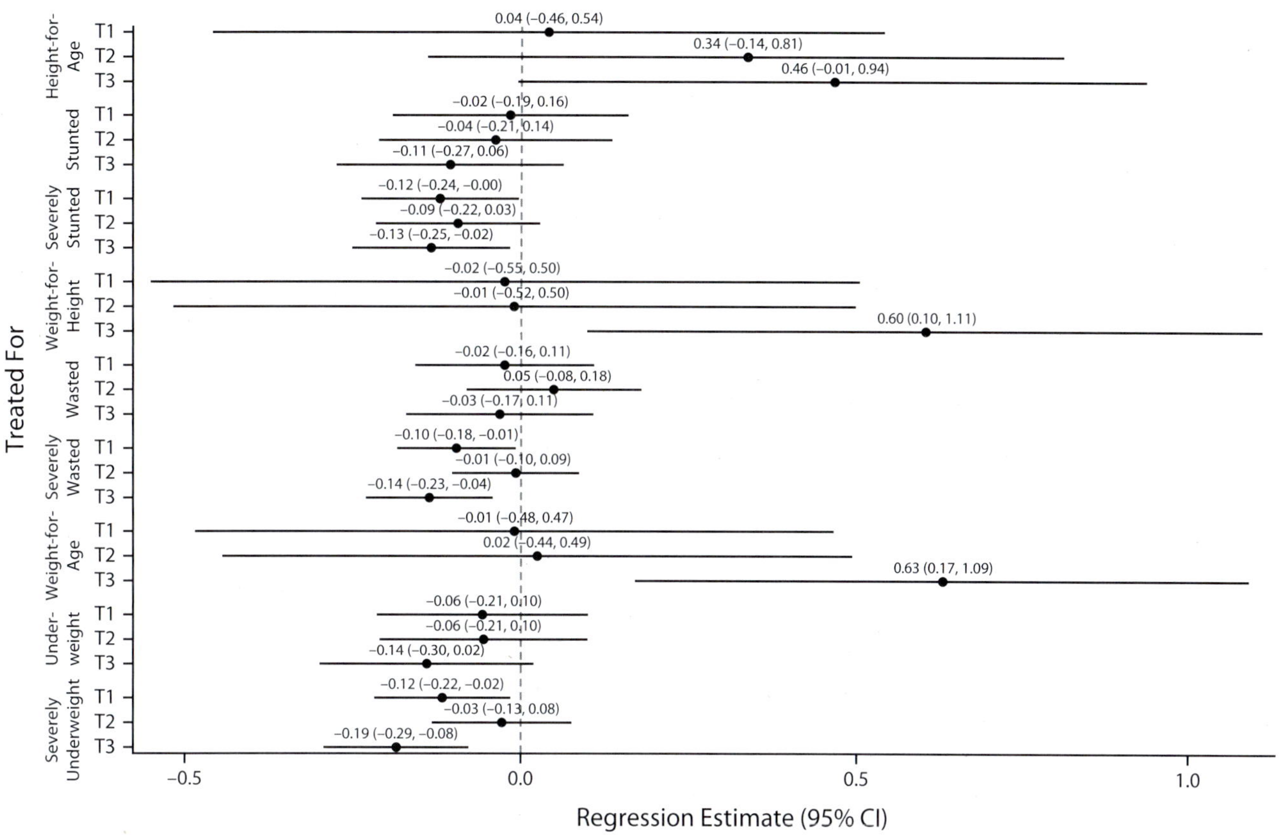

FIGURE 3— **Disaggregated Treatment Heterogeneity Analysis for Male Children (Effects Additional to Those for Female Children): Pakistan, September–October 2021**

Note. CI = confidence interval; T1 = monthly in-home growth monitoring with counseling (IHGMC); T2 = IHGMC with a poster-sized HAZ (height-for-age *z*-score)–based growth monitoring interactive chart; T3 = IHGMC plus growth charts (as in T2) complemented with a monthly unconditional cash transfer.

reported improved gender-related attitudes toward care, an increase of 0.17 SD (95% CI = 0.01, 0.32; *P* = .04) in a standardized index for multiple categories of child care–related questions, a larger quantity of fish and meat (0.10 SD; 95% CI = 0.02, 0.19; *P* = .02), and a greater dietary diversity score (0.35 SD; 95% CI = −0.01, 0.72; *P* = .06). However, we note that caregivers in this arm also demonstrated a 0.22 SD decrease (95% CI = −0.38, −0.05; *P* = .01) in general health care knowledge.

DISCUSSION

Our study has 3 major results. First, ours is one of the first studies demonstrating the impact of regular IHGMC by CHWs on young children, and we found a 0.42 SD gain in HAZ. To put this estimate into perspective, a range of comparable studies found increases in HAZ that did not exceed 0.25 SD, with time horizons ranging from a few months to 2 years.[20,26–28] This is an important finding because gains in height are harder to achieve and represent a relatively permanent positive change in health, unlike weight, which tends to respond quicker to a range of inputs. The gains in height that we documented are especially significant because these were realized during the COVID-19 pandemic, when income shocks resulted in severe nutritional deficiency in poor countries.[4] Our sample suffered aggregate welfare and health shocks; 75% of our sample reported that a member of the household lost work and 76% reported a loss in income due to the pandemic.

Second, we found that the simple IHGMC intervention contributed the most to child anthropometric outcomes. Specifically, we found that having IHGMC alone (T1) resulted in a 0.58 SD gain in HAZ, but layering a growth chart and unconditional cash transfer on top of IHGMC yielded positive albeit lower gains in child health. This suggests that the growth charts added complexity that resulted in these relatively lower gains. In our endline survey—7 months after the intervention—we specifically asked whether the growth chart was still in use and its primary function was understood. Use of the growth chart was not universal in the treatment groups; households reported limited use (14%) of the growth chart in the postintervention period. Moreover, they had questionable understanding of the chart; 60% failed to explain how the chart worked. These facts suggest that more effort may be needed from CHWs in explaining the growth charts to primary caregivers for greater understanding and usability.

Third, we found that the cash arm (T3) had a gendered effect: male children in the cash transfer arm differentially benefited on almost all anthropometric measures. Male children in T3 had higher HAZ, WAZ, and WHZ scores and lower probability of being severely stunted, severely wasted, underweight, or severely underweight. The simple IHGMC and the IHGMC with growth chart, however, did not show a gendered effect. These facts suggest that the simplest intervention of IHGMC tends to work equally well for children, irrespective of gender. Moreover, any program that chooses to add cash transfers must carefully consider gender dynamics in their respective settings. Our study showed that the cash transfer differentially benefited male children; this may be a consequence of local cultural preferences, including son bias.[29] Additional programming and counseling are needed to encourage more gender-equal allocation of resources.

Our results have several implications. First, we have demonstrated the effectiveness of a relatively simple intervention to induce gains in child height and weight by providing monthly nutrition counseling and in-home growth monitoring through direct engagement of caregivers by CHWs. Second, we effectively served households in an informal urban settlement. These communities are typically underserved, having few formal high-quality health facilities—which was exacerbated during the COVID-19 pandemic. Third, our program has the potential for scale in dense urban settings where homes are close to each other and CHWs do not need to carry equipment for long distances. We followed the established CHW model that orients the IHGMC intervention for the possibility of scaling-up with other CHW programs, which abound across the developing world. Our program is cost-effective: the total monthly cost of implementation per child in the IHGMC arm (T1) was $18 (including intervention, implementation, and administrative costs); the cost per case of stunting averted by the intervention was $360 (total implementation cost divided by additional cases of stunting averted in T1 compared with the control), which is on the lower end of the range for similar interventions in Pakistan and globally ($202–$1107).

Our study has 3 limitations. First, we noticed sizable attrition of our sample with unequal survey retention propensity across the treatment groups (Table A13 of online Appendix A). This is a consequence of working in informal settlement areas, which challenged our logistical capability. Working in an urban informal settlement is difficult[28,30] because there are no formal addresses and many dwellers tend to out-migrate (average annual turnovers of 25% have been documented). On the basis of information from key informants, we understood that this high rate of out-migration is reasonable, as the community is predominantly Pashtun immigrants who are highly mobile and frequently change address. Second, this reduced sample likely affected our ability to detect statistically significant differences in subgroup analysis. Finally, our treatment assignment was at the household level. Despite the highly idiosyncratic nature of our program, which delivered household-specific counseling and made child-specific measurements, households in our treatment group may have shared some insights from their experiences with households in their network. This has the potential to produce a positive spillover effect by contaminating the treatment and control groups, making the impact estimates lower bounds.

Taken together, we have demonstrated that a simple, low-cost, scalable intervention—regular home-based growth monitoring and nutrition counseling by CHWs—has a sizable impact on child HAZ and associated reduction in severe stunting, measured during the COVID-19 pandemic. Our findings suggest that regular IHGMC can increase resilience to malnutrition. These are compelling findings, in terms of tackling both the long-term challenge of child stunting and the short-term impact during this global pandemic, and they provide an important policy tool for low- and middle-income countries. AJPH

ABOUT THE AUTHORS

Abu S. Shonchoy is with the Department of Economics, Steven J. Green School of International and Public Affairs, Florida International University, Miami. At the time of this work, Agha A. Akram was with the Department of Economics, Mushtaq Ahmad Gurmani School of Social Science, Lahore University of Management Sciences; Mahrukh Khan was with the Centre for Economic Research in Pakistan; Hina Khalid was with the Department of Economics, School of Humanities and Social Sciences, Information Technology University; and Sidra Mazhar was with the Center for Economic Research in Pakistan, Lahore, Pakistan. Akib Khan is with the Department of Economics, Uppsala University, Uppsala, Sweden. Takashi Kurosaki is with the Institute of Economic Research, Hitotsubashi University, Tokyo, Japan.

CORRESPONDENCE

Correspondence should be sent to Abu S. Shonchoy, Florida International University, 11200 SW 8th St,

Miami, FL 33199 (e-mail: shonchoy@fiu.edu).
Reprints can be ordered at http://www.ajph.org by clicking the "Reprints" link.

PUBLICATION INFORMATION

Full Citation: Shonchoy AS, Akram AA, Khan M, et al. A community health worker–based intervention on anthropometric outcomes of children aged 3 to 21 months in urban Pakistan, 2019–2021. *Am J Public Health*. 2023;113(1):105–114.

Acceptance Date: August 29, 2022.

DOI: https://doi.org/10.2105/AJPH.2022.307111

CONTRIBUTORS

A. S. Shonchoy conceptualized the research idea, conducted the formal analysis, acquired funding, designed the methodology, and guided the analysis; he administered and supervised the implementation of this study, was involved in the writing of the original draft, and led the revision of the article. A. A. Akram conceptualized the research idea, conducted the formal analysis, acquired funding, designed the methodology, and guided the analysis; he administered and supervised the implementation of this study, managed resources, was involved in the writing of the original draft, and led revision of the article. M. Khan curated the data set, conducted the formal analysis, and managed project resources and the software for analysis; she conducted the data validation, created visualizations, and was involved in the writing of the original draft and the revisions of the article. H. Khalid conducted the formal analysis, acquired funding, designed the methodology, and guided the analysis; she administered and supervised the project and was involved in the writing of the original draft and the revisions of the article. S. Mazhar conducted the investigation, administered the project, and participated in data validation; she was also involved in the writing of the original draft of the article. A. Khan conceptualized the research idea, conducted the formal analysis, acquired funding, designed the methodology, and guided the analysis; he administered and supervised the project, managed project resources and the software, led the data validation and analysis, and was involved in the writing of the original draft of the article. T. Kurosaki conducted the formal analysis, acquired funding, designed the methodology, and led the investigation; he also supervised the implementation of this study, and was involved in the writing of the original draft and the revisions of the article.

ACKNOWLEDGMENTS

We are grateful to the Center for Economic Research in Pakistan for research support and Sukoon Water for implementation support. Our sincere gratitude goes to our funders for funding our research: the World Bank, the Shahid Hussain Foundation, Lahore University of Management Sciences, and Hitotsubashi University.

We received useful feedback on our manuscript from Nathan Congdon, Jocelyn Finley, Ashley Fox, Alaka Holla, Ghazala Mansuri, Atonu Rabbani, Kanako Yamashita-Allen, Aisha Yousufzai, Mazvita Zanamwe, and the conference participants of the Southern Economic Association Conference in 2020.

CONFLICTS OF INTEREST

We declare that we have no conflicts of interest.

HUMAN PARTICIPANT PROTECTION

Ethical approval to conduct this study was obtained from the institutional review board at Interactive Research and Development (Karachi approval no. IRD_IRB_2018_09_003). Oral consent was obtained from all caregivers before the survey was administered.

REFERENCES

1. de Onis M, Blössner M, Borghi E. Prevalence and trends of stunting among pre-school children, 1990–2020. *Public Health Nutr*. 2012;15(1):142–148. https://doi.org/10.1017/S1368980011001315
2. UNICEF. Nutrition, for every child: UNICEF Nutrition Strategy 2020–2030. 2020. Available at: https://www.unicef.org/media/92031/file/UNICEF%20Nutrition%20Strategy%202020-2030.pdf. Accessed November 8, 2022.
3. Prendergast A, Humphrey J. The stunting syndrome in developing countries. *Paediatr Int Child Health*. 2014;34(4):250–265. https://doi.org/10.1179/2046905514Y.0000000158
4. Egger D, Miguel E, Warren S, et al. Falling living standards during the COVID-19 crisis: quantitative evidence from nine developing countries. *Sci Adv*. 2021;7(6):eabe0997. https://doi.org/10.1126/sciadv.abe0997
5. Headey D, Heidkamp R, Osendarp S, et al. Impacts of COVID-19 on childhood malnutrition and nutrition-related mortality. *Lancet*. 2020;396(10250):519–521. https://doi.org/10.1016/S0140-6736(20)31647-0
6. Fore H, Dongyu Q, Beasley D, Ghebreyesus T. Child malnutrition and COVID-19: the time to act is now. *Lancet*. 2020;396(10250):517–518. https://doi.org/10.1016/S0140-6736(20)31648-2
7. Dept of Child and Adolescent Health and Development. *The Importance of Caregiver–Child Interactions for the Survival and Healthy Development of Young Children*. Geneva, Switzerland: World Health Organization; 2004. Available at: https://www.who.int/publications/i/item/924159134X. Accessed November 14, 2022.
8. Mistry S, Hossain M, Arora A. Maternal nutrition counselling is associated with reduced stunting prevalence and improved feeding practices in early childhood: a post-program comparison study. *Nutr J*. 2019;18(1):47. https://doi.org/10.1186/s12937-019-0473-z
9. Yousafzai A, Obradović J, Rasheed M, et al. Effects of responsive stimulation and nutrition interventions on children's development and growth at age 4 years in a disadvantaged population in Pakistan: a longitudinal follow-up of a cluster-randomised factorial effectiveness trial. *Lancet Glob Health*. 2016;4(8):e548–e558. https://doi.org/10.1016/S2214-109X(16)30100-0
10. Perry HB, Hodgins S. Health for the people: past, current, and future contributions of national community health worker programs to achieving global health goals. *Glob Health Sci Pract*. 2021;9(1):1–9. https://doi.org/10.9745/GHSP-D-20-00459
11. Vaivada T, Akseer N, Akseer S, Somaskandan A, Stefopulos M, Bhutta Z. Stunting in childhood: an overview of global burden, trends, determinants, and drivers of decline. *Am J Clin Nutr*. 2020;112(suppl 2):777S–791S. https://doi.org/10.1093/ajcn/nqaa159
12. Ashworth A, Shrimpton R, Jamil K. Growth monitoring and promotion: review of evidence of impact. *Matern Child Nutr*. 2008;4(suppl 1):86–117. https://doi.org/10.1111/j.1740-8709.2007.00125.x
13. Galasso E, Weber A, Stewart C, Ratsifandrihamanana L, Fernald L. Effects of nutritional supplementation and home visiting on growth and development in young children in Madagascar: a cluster-randomised controlled trial. *Lancet Glob Health*. 2019;7(9):e1257–e1268. https://doi.org/10.1016/S2214-109X(19)30317-1
14. Swarthout J, Ram P, Arnold C, et al. Effects of individual and combined water, sanitation, handwashing, and nutritional interventions on child respiratory infections in rural Kenya: a cluster-randomized controlled trial. *Am J Trop Med Hyg*. 2020;102(6):1286–1295. https://doi.org/10.4269/ajtmh.19-0779
15. Kim K, Choi J, Choi E, et al. Effects of community-based health worker interventions to improve chronic disease management and care among vulnerable populations: a systematic review. *Am J Public Health*. 2016;106(4):e3–e28. https://doi.org/10.2105/AJPH.2015.302987
16. Manley J, Balarajan Y, Malm S, et al. Cash transfers and child nutritional outcomes: a systematic review and meta-analysis. *BMJ Glob Health*. 2020;5(12):e003621. https://doi.org/10.1136/bmjgh-2020-003621
17. Ruel M, Alderman H. Nutrition-sensitive interventions and programmes: how can they help to accelerate progress in improving maternal and child nutrition? *Lancet*. 2013;382(9891):536–551. https://doi.org/10.1016/S0140-6736(13)60843-0
18. George S, Latham M, Frongillo E, Abel R, Ethirajan N. Evaluation of effectiveness of good growth monitoring in south Indian villages. *Lancet*. 1993;342(8867):348–352. https://doi.org/10.1016/0140-6736(93)91479-6
19. Shekar M, Latham M. Growth monitoring can and does work! An example from the Tamil Nadu Integrated Nutrition Project in rural South India. *Indian J Pediatr*. 1992;59(1):5–15. https://doi.org/10.1007/BF02760889
20. Fink G, Levenson R, Tembo S, Rockers P. Home- and community-based growth monitoring to reduce early life growth faltering: an open-label, cluster-randomized controlled trial. *Am J Clin Nutr*. 2017;106(4):1070–1077. https://doi.org/10.3945/ajcn.117.157545
21. National Institute of Population Studies (NIPS) [Pakistan] and Inner City Fund International Inc (ICF). *Pakistan Demographic and Health Survey 2017–18*. Rockville, MD: NIPS and ICF; 2019.
22. UNICEF. Impact of Covid-19 on children living in poverty. Available at: https://data.unicef.org/topic/nutrition/child-nutrition-and-covid-19. Accessed December 24, 2021.
23. Iacus S, King G, Porro G. Causal inference without balance checking: coarsened exact matching. *Polit Anal*. 2012;20(1):1–24. https://doi.org/10.1093/pan/mpr013
24. World Health Organization. Child growth standards. 2021. Available at: https://www.who.int/

tools/child-growth-standards. Accessed December 24, 2021.

25. de Onis M. Development of a WHO growth reference for school-aged children and adolescents. *Bull World Health Organ.* 2007;85(9):660–667. https://doi.org/10.2471/BLT.07.043497
26. Roy SK, Fuchs GJ, Mahmud Z, et al. Intensive nutrition education with or without supplementary feeding improves the nutritional status of moderately-malnourished children in Bangladesh. *J Health Popul Nutr.* 2005;23(4):320–330.
27. Zaman S, Ashraf RN, Martines J. Training in complementary feeding counselling of healthcare workers and its influence on maternal behaviours and child growth: a cluster-randomized controlled trial in Lahore, Pakistan. *J Health Popul Nutr.* 2008;26(2):210–222.
28. Rains E, Krishna A, Webbels E. *Urbanisation and India's Slum Continuum: Evidence on the Range of Policy Needs and Scope of Mobility.* London, UK: International Growth Center; 2018.
29. Jayachandran S, Pande R. Why are Indian children so short? The role of birth order and son preference. *Am Econ Rev.* 2017;107(9):2600–2629. https://doi.org/10.1257/aer.20151282
30. Krishna A, Sriram M, Prakash P. Slum types and adaptation strategies: identifying policy-relevant differences in Bangalore. *Environ Urban.* 2014; 26(2):568–585. https://doi.org/10.1177/0956247814537958

Trends in Degree Conferrals, Degree-Associated Debt, and Employment Outcomes Among Undergraduate Public Health Degree Graduates, 2001–2020

Jonathon P. Leider, PhD, Emily Burke, EdD, MPH, CPH, Ruby H. N. Nguyen, PhD, MHS, Christine Plepys, MS, Chelsey Kirkland, PhD, MPH, CHW, Beth Resnick, DrPH, MPH, and Laura Magaña, PhD, MS

See also Riegelman, p. 9.

Objectives. To characterize the trends in degree conferrals, degree-associated debt, and employment outcomes among undergraduate public health degree (UGPHD) graduates.

Methods. We reported administrative data on degree conferrals from 2001 to 2020 from the National Center for Education Statistics (NCES). For alumni graduating from 2015 to 2019, we also reported degree-associated debt and earnings 1 year after graduation compiled by NCES. Finally, we utilized a data set on 1-year postgraduation employment outcomes for graduates from 2015 to 2020 from the Association of Schools and Programs of Public Health.

Results. As of 2020, more than 18 000 UGPHDs were awarded each year, more than 140 000 in total over the past 20 years. UGPHD graduates are highly diverse, with more than 80% being women and 55% being individuals from communities of color. We find alumni worked mostly in for-profit organizations (34%), health care (28%), nonprofits (11%), academic organizations (10%), government (10%), and other (6%). Degree-associated debt was $24 000, and the median first-year earnings were $34 000.

Conclusions. While growth in UGPHD conferrals has slowed, it remains among the fastest-growing degree in the nation. However, the limited pathways into government remains a significant challenge. (*Am J Public Health*. 2023;113(1):115–123. https://doi.org/10.2105/AJPH.2022.307113)

AJPH January 2023, Vol 113, No. 1

The undergraduate public health degree (UGPHD) surpassed the master's degree in 2020 as the most conferred public health degree in the United States.[1] This rapid growth began in 2004, fueled in part by the rise in bioterrorism concerns and interest in strengthening the nation's public health system in the aftermath of 9/11 and the 2001 anthrax attacks.[2] The growth was also fueled by the seminal work published in the 2003 Institute of Medicine report recommending that all undergraduates have access to education in public health and the proliferation of accredited graduate schools and programs of public health.[3] More than twice the number of undergraduate students graduated with public health degrees from 2008 to 2012 than from 1992 to 2008, and the majority of students graduated with UGPHDs in general public health and health education or behavioral sciences.[4,5] It is also a degree whose recipients are far more racially and ethnically diverse than recipients of graduate degrees in general.[5] Yet, despite this marked growth, the UGPHD is once again in transition.

Degree conferrals have been driven both by growth within existing programs and by new entrants to the marketplace.[4,5] About 271 institutions offered UGPHDs in 2016 compared with 179 in 2012, with about 50% coming from institutions with public health degree programs that were accredited by the Council on Education for Public Health (CEPH).[5,6] CEPH was established in 1974 to serve as the independent accreditation body for graduate schools and programs of public health.[7] CEPH's standalone baccalaureate accreditation was introduced in 2016; there are currently 25 standalone CEPH-accredited baccalaureate programs.[8] The expansion of standalone programs is indicative of an expanded breadth of programs without other master's-level public health training.[6] Furthermore, this new accreditation offers the opportunity to greatly expand the reach of public health education to other institutions across the country and to increase diversity both in student populations and geographic regions.[6]

Before this effort, UGPHD programs were only accredited if they were conferred by a CEPH-accredited graduate school of public health. However, now, with the drastic increase in undergraduate public health program offerings and with the number of UGPHDs conferred, several key questions have arisen regarding the UGPHD. Questions include the potential role of the UGPHD on the field's ability to diversify the public health workforce, establish pathways for training, reduce overlap with the graduate-level curriculum, and ultimately rebuild the governmental public health workforce with new UGPHD graduates.[1]

Especially of note are the employment outcomes for bachelor's students, including both what types of jobs they would get in general and, specifically, whether those jobs would substitute for master's-trained alumni, as had happened in other fields in previous decades.[1,3,9,10] For example, there is a current debate about whether hospitals should hire a certified registered nurse anesthetist or an anesthesiologist, with the former being less expensive, yet debate on cost-effectiveness and ultimate practice models remains.[11,12]

Given these questions, as well as the recent increased limelight on public health as a result of the COVID-19 pandemic, in this study, we explored recent trends in public health undergraduate education with a focus on first-destination outcomes, including employment or further higher education, of UGPHD recipients.

METHODS

We used 3 data sets to characterize the UGPHD trends in the United States: the Integrated Postsecondary Education Data System (IPEDS),[13] the College Scorecard from the National Center for Education Statistics (NCES), and first-destination outcomes from the Association of Schools and Programs of Public Health (ASPPH).[14]

Our research utilized IPEDS data that catalogued degree conferrals for UGPHD programs in the United States that were reported from 2001 through 2020. IPEDS data are reported annually by all public and private postsecondary institutions that receive federal support, including federally backed financial aid. Degree conferral data are one of several required reporting areas, which also include enrollments, admissions, academic offerings, salary spending on faculty and staff, and staff composition, among other organizational characteristics.

IPEDS maintains data on institutional characteristics for each college or university in its data set; of primary interest are institutional (Carnegie) classification, control institution (public, private not-for-profit, private for-profit), and geographic region. UGPHD programs were identified with Classification of Instructional Program (CIP) codes (National Center for Education Statistics, https://bit.ly/3gCEbHC), including for public health (CIP 51.22XX), as well as for health policy analysis (44.0503), epidemiology (26.1309), and biostatistics (26.1102), which IPEDS classifies outside of public health (Table A, available as a supplement to the online version of this article at https://ajph.org). While NCES does not include biostatistics, epidemiology, or health policy, they have long been included as core degrees or program offers in public health institutions. IPEDS data before 2010 are crosswalked to the 2020 CIP code standards.

NCES constructs estimates of earnings and degree-associated debt using federal administrative data and publishes these data annually via the College Scorecard. These estimates are reported by institution, degree, degree level, and 4-digit CIP code family. NCES constructs these estimates by 2-year cohorts, with earnings information drawn from Internal Revenue Service filings of graduates 1 year after graduation and degree-associated debt from Free Application for Federal Student Aid filings. Data were available on students graduating in 2015 through 2019 at the time of this analysis, in spring 2022. NCES notes that institution-level data may be censored if there are insufficient student record matches or number of graduates. NCES data are thought to constitute the universe of public health degree conferrals in the United States but do not include first-destination outcomes.

The third data set was provided by ASPPH. Since 2016, ASPPH has collected first-destination outcomes data through its membership, CEPH-accredited schools and programs of public health in the United States and abroad (only domestic data were used in this analysis). Students who are graduating, and up to 1 year after graduation, report first-destination outcomes to their schools and programs of public health. These data are de-identified and reported to ASPPH. Among those reporting employment outcomes, both broad employment sector and detailed sector are reported. The most recent available data are from graduating years 2015 through 2020 (collected up to 1 year later) and are included in this assessment.

ASPPH data include graduates of UGPHD programs at accredited schools and programs of public health, which represent approximately 48% of graduates from UGPHD programs in the United States captured in IPEDS data. Please see Figure A (available as a supplement to the online version of this article at https://ajph.org) for the number of applicants to MPH programs in Schools of Public Health Application Service, the centralized application service, by major or concentration in undergraduate degrees.

We calculated descriptive statistics to report findings from the administrative data sources. We used Stata version 17.1 (StataCorp LLC, College Station, TX) and Tableau Desktop (Tableau Software, Mountain View, CA) for analysis.

RESULTS

In 2001, colleges and universities across the United States reported awarding 1480 UGPHDs, compared with 5576 graduate public health degrees. By 2020, 18 289 UGPHDs and 19 641 graduate public health degrees (18 044 and 1597 master's and doctorate degrees, respectively) had been awarded (Figure 1). The UGPHD grew an average 13.4% each year over the past 2 decades, eventually eclipsing the master's degree as the most conferred public health degree type in the United States in 2020.

Demographics of Degree Grantors and Recipients

The number of institutions awarding solely UGPHDs with no graduate public health degrees has also grown substantially, from 44 in 2001 to 183 in 2020. As of 2020, more than 550 institutions awarded either a UGPHD or graduate public health degrees, with 392 awarding at least 1 UGPHD and 265 institutions awarding at least 10 UGPHDs. In terms of the size of graduating classes by institution, the median was 20 degrees conferred in 2020, with the 25th percentile at 7 degrees and the 75th percentile at 55 degrees. Between 2001 and 2020, 143 000 UGPHD conferrals were captured by NCES, of which about 24 000 were conferred between 2001 and 2010, 35 000

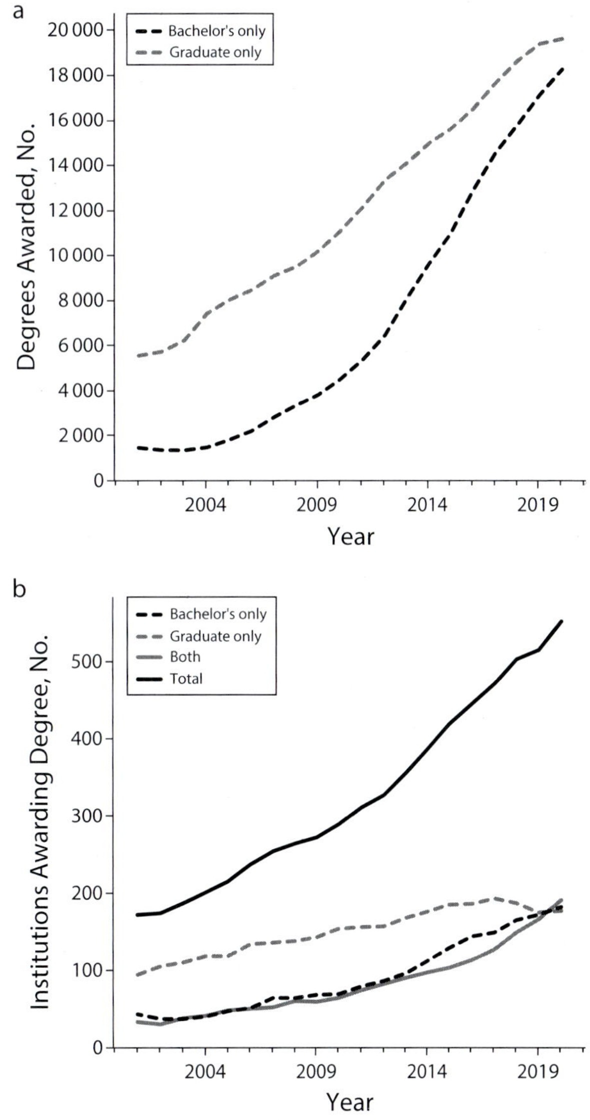

FIGURE 1— Number of (a) Public Health Degrees Awarded and (b) Degree-Awarding Institutions: United States, 2001–2020

between 2011 and 2015, and 79 000 between 2016 and 2020.

Data from NCES show wide racial and ethnic diversity of UGPHD graduates. In 2020, 45% were White. Hispanic/Latino students constituted the second-largest group of graduates (17%), followed by Black/African American (15%), Asian (13%), 2 or more race (4%), and American Indian/Alaska Native (1%) students. International students represented 2.5% of UGPHD conferrals, and another 2.5% of graduates had unknown race/ethnicity status. Women constituted 80% of conferrals in 2020, an increase from 69% in 2001.

Compared with graduate public health degree conferrals, during the past 2 decades, a smaller percentage of undergraduates received their UGPHD from a CEPH-accredited school or program of public health (Figure 2). Coincident with CEPH instituting a standalone undergraduate accreditation standard in 2016 (and therefore affording accreditation to students graduating up to 3 years before[15]), the majority of UGPHDs were conferred by a CEPH-accredited school or program of public health or a standalone baccalaureate program. In 2020, 57% of UGPHDs came from CEPH-accredited institutions and programs, compared with 82% of master's degrees and 89% of doctoral degrees. We observed differences by race/ethnicity; 74% of Asian students received a UGPHD in 2020 from a CEPH-accredited institution and programs, compared with 56% of Black students, 53% of Hispanic/Latino students, and 55% of White students. We similarly observed differences in graduation by control of institution (public, private not-for-profit, or private for-profit) by race/ethnicity.

Conferrals by type of institution changed substantially since 2001, when 88% of UGPHDs came from public institutions, 11% from private not-for-profit, and less than 1% from private for-profit. In 2020, 75% of UGPHD conferrals came from public institutions, 22% from private not-for-profit, and 3% from for-profit institutions. In 2020, among Asian students, less than 1% of UGPHDs came from for-profit institutions, as did 9% of UGPHDs earned by Black students, 4% earned by Hispanic/Latino students, and 2% earned by White students.

First-Destination Outcomes

Among 23 810 UGPHD graduates between 2015 and 2020 with first-destination outcomes reported to ASPPH, 7% reported seeking employment, 31% reported enrollment in further study, and 62% reported having employment, a fellowship, or a volunteer position. Among the 8724 UGPHD graduates with full-time employment outcomes reported, 34% reported working within for-profit organizations, 28% in health care

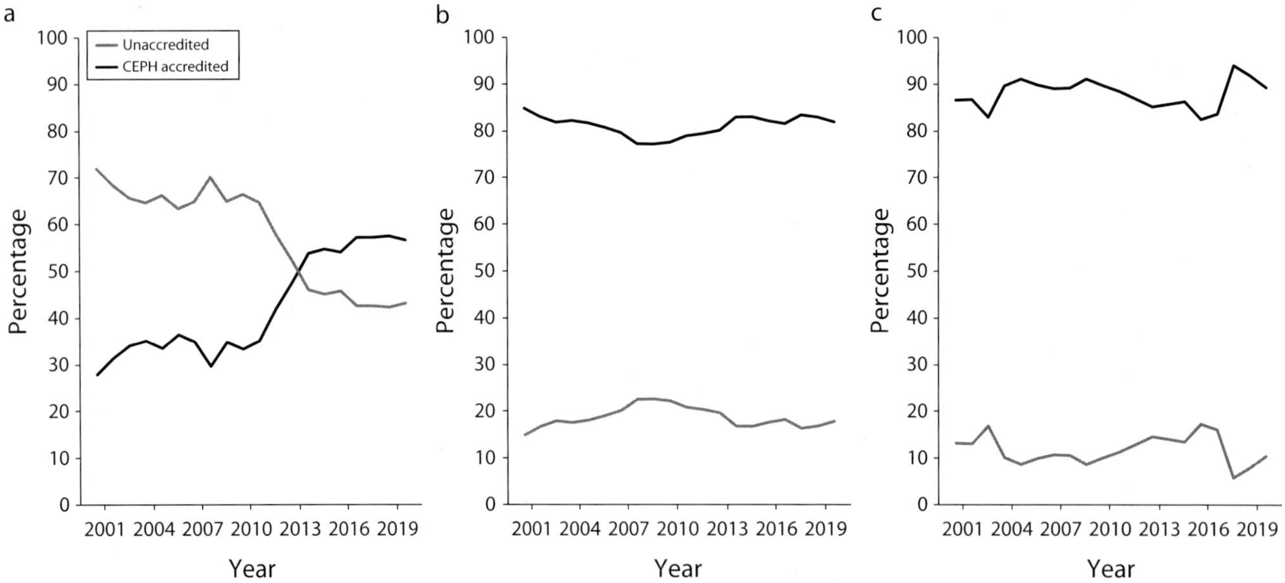

FIGURE 2— Public Health Degrees Awarded, by Accreditation Status and Percentage of (a) Bachelor's Degrees, (b) Master's Degrees, and (c) Doctoral Degrees: United States, 2001–2020

Note. CEPH = Council on Education for Public Health.

organizations, 11% in nonprofit organizations, 10% in academic institutions, 10% in government, and 6% in "other" (Figure 3).

Detailed employment-sector information was provided by 10 939 UGPHD graduates. Of those working in academic institutions, two thirds worked in postsecondary education and one quarter in K–12 education. Among those working in for-profit organizations, 13% worked in consulting; 16% in marketing, public relations, communications, and pharmaceuticals; and 8% in health insurance and information technology. Among those in government positions, 24% worked in federal, 26% in state, 38% in local, 9% in military, and 3% in "other types." Of those working in the health care sector, 36% reported being within hospital and health systems and 6% in managed care.

Lastly, for UGPHD graduates who reported pursuing further study, 36% were pursuing a graduate public health degree, 27% were pursuing a medical or clinical degree, and 37% were pursuing another or unknown degree.

NCES publishes degree-associated debt and postgraduation earnings through their College Scorecard (Figure 4). Median degree-associated debt for students graduating in 2014 to 2019 was highest among for-profit institutions awarding UGPHDs (median = $39 800; interquartile range [IQR] = $39 000–$42 000), compared with not-for-profit institutions (median = $26 000; IQR = $23 000–$27 000) and public institutions (median = $22 000; IQR = $19 000–$25 000). One-year postgraduation earnings data were comparable across all institution types (median = approximately $34 000). Median degree-associated debt and earnings varied widely for UGPHDs by geographic region, with degree-associated debt being highest in the mid-east and New England regions, and lowest in Rocky Mountain and far-west regions. Median 1-year postgraduation earnings ranged from $31 000 to $38 000 with the lowest being from the southeast region and highest from New England.

DISCUSSION

In 2020, nearly 20 000 UGPHDs were conferred. While UGPHDs have overtaken master's degrees as the most-awarded public health degrees in the United States, accredited master's degree conferrals still substantially outnumber accredited undergraduate degrees. This is not surprising given IPEDS reporting indicates that 89% of doctoral and 82% of master's degrees were conferred by universities with a

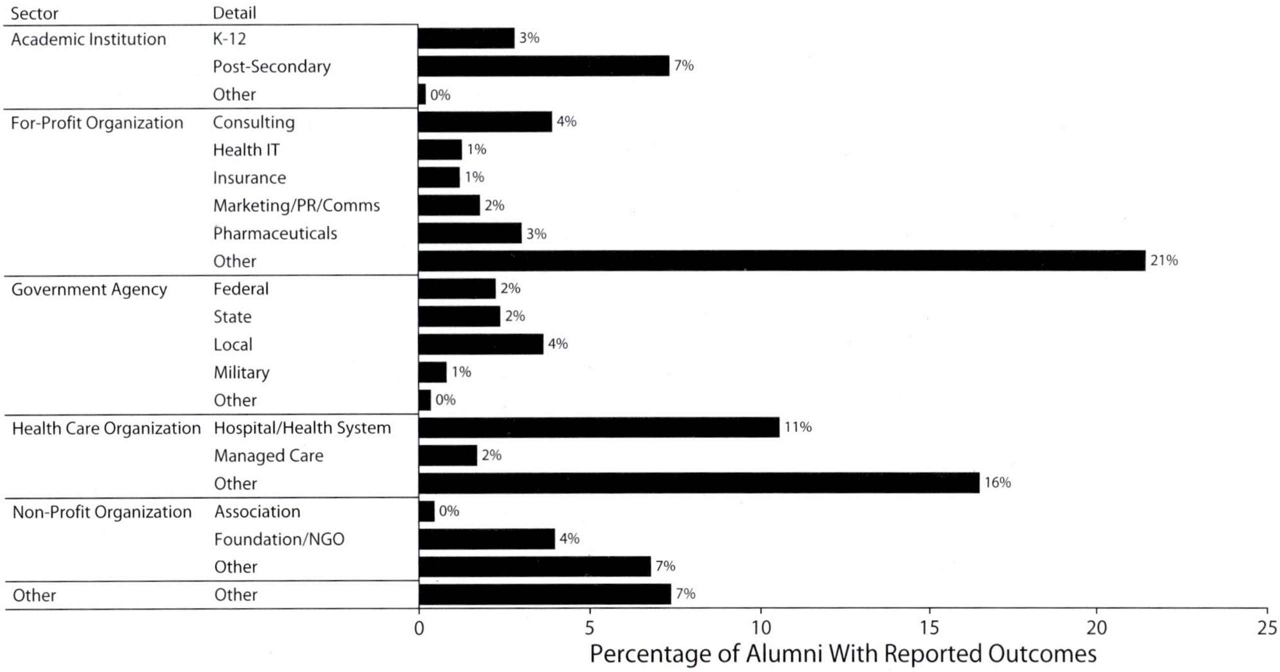

FIGURE 3— First-Destination Employment Outcomes by Sector Among Undergraduate Public Health Degree Alumni, Graduating Years 2015–2020: United States

Note. IT = information technology; NGO = nongovernmental organization; PR = public relations. Figure shows median earnings by institution. Listed percentages are rounded to the nearest whole number.

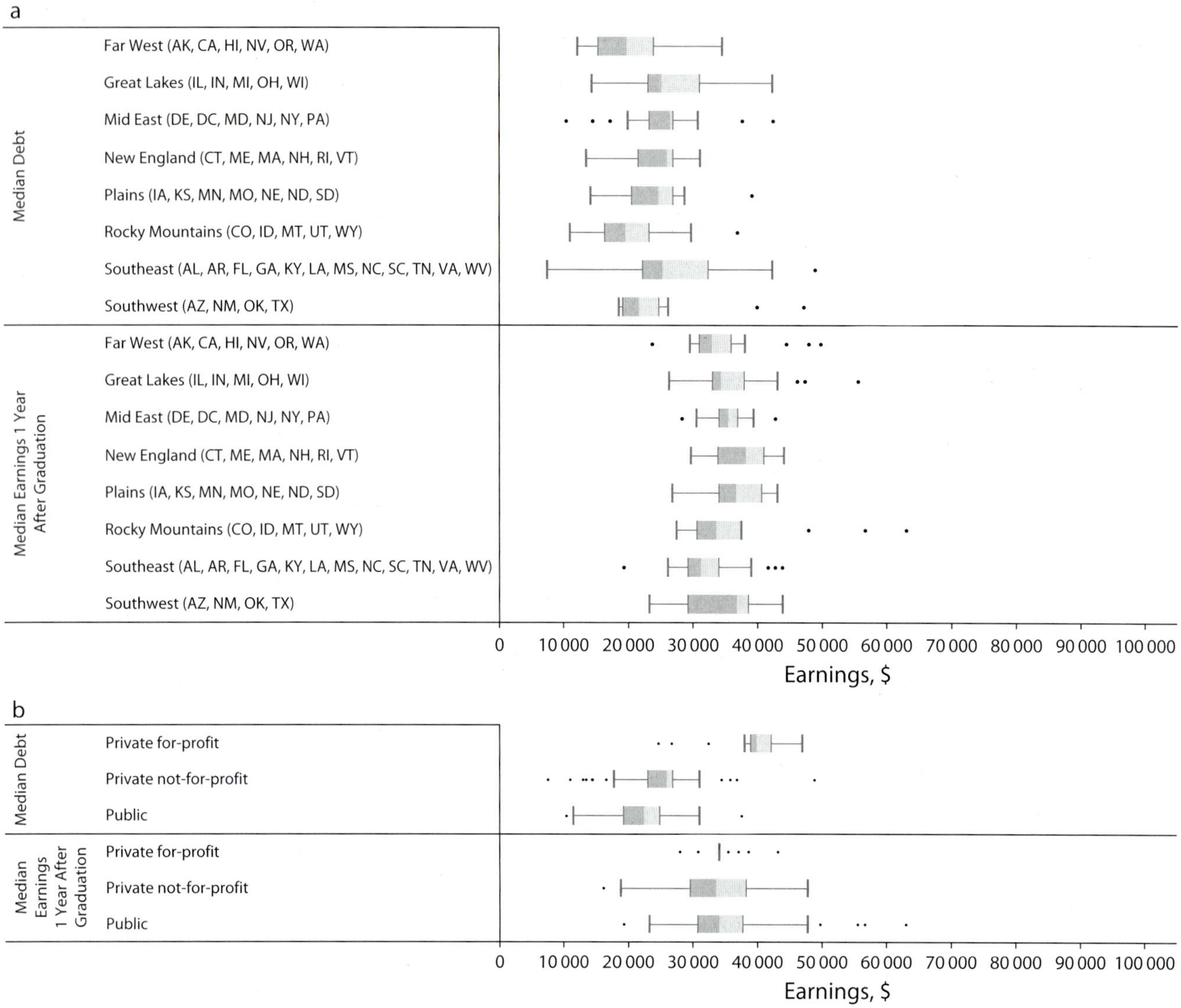

FIGURE 4— Earnings 1 Year After Graduation and Degree-Associated Debt Among Undergraduate Public Health Degree Alumni by (a) Bureau of Economic Analysis Region and (b) Control of Institution: United States, Graduating Years 2014–2019

CEPH-accredited schools and programs of public health while only 57% of UGPHDs were conferred by a university with a CEPH-accredited public health school, program, or standalone baccalaureate program.

UGPHD graduates secure employment in multiple industries upon graduation, and many pursue further higher education, including graduate studies in public health. Of those graduates securing employment, relatively few have pursued a job in governmental public health (10%), while the majority (62%) enter the workforce in the for-profit sector or in the health care sector. This differs somewhat from graduate program alumni, where 17% have pursued jobs in governmental public health and 41% landed in the for-profit or health care sector. Further more, the percentage of graduate program alumni working in governmental public health has increased each year since ASPPH began collecting first destinations outcomes data, with 21% of master's and doctoral graduates entering the governmental public health workforce in 2020.[16] This might suggest that UGPHD and graduate alumni are not competing for the same jobs as has been previously hypothesized.

However, it is reasonable, if not prudent, for public health practitioners to concretely distinguish job tasks and desired skills of undergraduates from graduates in the workplace while academic public health better communicates the continuum and progressive nature of the competencies that graduates demonstrate at the undergraduate, master's, and doctoral level.[9,17] These distinctions would ensure undergraduates and graduates do not compete for the same position and limit the ongoing concern about the threat of a "substitution effect," in which baccalaureate degree holders are preferentially hired at lower wages for the same jobs that graduate degree-holders had been previously recruited, in the government sector (or elsewhere). The concern arises from a history in other fields.[4,5,9,17] The best way to ensure a substitution effect does not occur is through task and skill differentiation for different levels of academic achievement.

We show that undergraduate public health is continuing to grow, that several hundred institutions are now offering these degrees, that graduates are pursuing a variety of jobs and sectors as employment outcomes, and that there is a wide range of earnings and debt loads associated with UGPHDs across the United States. Heterogeneity in UGPHDs, and education more broadly, is to be expected, even in an accredited field. In some respects, education is a marketplace, not just of ideas, but also one based on consumer and employer interests and needs, as well as one in which competition rewards positive program outcomes. A breadth of public health offerings should be encouraged, if they are indeed identifiable as public health programs.[17]

Institutions of higher education, in our view, should hold to core tenets of academic rigor and integrity and the pursuit of knowledge. At the same time, public health degrees are traditionally viewed in the vein of a professional degree, even at the undergraduate level, even where it is offered in the context of more general humanities or liberal arts programs. Fundamentally, after all, UGPHDs must be competency- and skill-based to be accreditable. There remains an open question about market saturation, especially considering continued and sustained growth, as well as broader opportunities for undergraduate public health–trained professionals to work in nontraditional areas, such as in public education, urban development, and political science. These remain substantive points for future discussion and research.

Reflections in Light of the Great Resignation

As we reflect on the future of undergraduate public health and its relationship to governmental public health, data presented in this article suggest that the United States may be approaching a point of opportunity. The governmental public health workforce is substantially depleted, generally since the Great Recession and specifically because of COVID-19 response (and the consequent Great Resignation/Reshuffling/Renegotiation).[18,19] Data recently released from the 2021 Public Health Workforce Interests and Needs Survey show 44% of staff are considering leaving their job or planning to retire within the next 5 years[20]; this represents more than 80 000 staff nationwide. Are public health graduates filling this gap? If not, who will?

Governmental public health has traditionally hired baccalaureate degree holders from other fields and some master's degree holders, the latter of whom sometimes have a UGPHD. Might this change with concerted efforts to create practice-based training programs and improve pathway development from the schools and programs of public health into government? Federal public health agencies have recognized the potential future gaps in the public health workforce and have established mechanisms to increase pipelines into governmental public health careers.[1,21–23]

These data suggest that now is a critical time for the initiation of partnerships between educational institutions and governmental public health agencies to better examine undergraduate public health education and to determine whether specific pathways to government are a priority and, if so, how then to implement them in ways that accomplish the desired aims. UGPHD recipients may serve health departments in key entry-level public health science and data-oriented positions. Yet, to attract these students away from health care, pharma, and for-profit firms, health departments must offer more efficient hiring processes, competitive wages and benefits, and clear opportunities for advancement, and seek to maximize engagement and perceptions of employee support within one's organization, as these factors are all key to recruitment and retention.[24,25]

A Matter of Demographics

A particular challenge undergraduate education faces broadly in the United States is the upcoming demographic cliff and the "Great Interruption" associated with COVID-19. As a result, in 2025 and beyond, fewer students are expected to graduate high school and enter college than in years past, though this has already begun in some regions.[26] There are simply fewer younger people seeking traditional bachelor's degrees (and, in turn, traditional master's), although there may be more midcareer professionals seeking further education. Further exacerbating this issue is the Great Interruption of COVID-19 whereby 21% fewer direct high school to college students enrolled in fall of 2020 when compared with 2019, and 1 in 4 college students failed to re-enroll in the fall of 2020.[27,28] In addition, uncertain macroeconomic conditions along with low unemployment rates may make college or graduate school less appealing.[29] These uncertain conditions will likely continue to be a concern for some time among institutions of higher education.

It is not clear to us what a broad decline in undergraduate enrollment might mean for a specific field such as public health. It may well be that in a postpandemic environment, public memory and interest in public health fade, and fewer undergraduates are aware of the public health degree. Conversely, because the next several years have dedicated federal public health infrastructure funding to grow pathways into governmental practice, schools and programs of public health may outcompete other resource-poor or otherwise flagging program areas for paid internships and better placement prospects out of school.

Even if undergraduate overall enrollment is down, public health enrollment could grow with appropriate strategy and investment such as using online education[30] and building and implementing an enrollment management plan.[31] This could be critical to rebuilding the governmental public health workforce and is especially relevant as enrollment in master's education in public health similarly in 2022 has begun again to slow down, likely attributable to degree-offering institution saturation, as had been projected for some time before the COVID-19–associated bump in admission.[32]

Limitations

When interpreting these trends, the following limitations should be considered. First, while the NCES is widely regarded as a reliable source of degree-conferral data,[32] misclassification may occur. Sensitivity analyses show that if institutions are excluded that conferred fewer than 10 undergraduate public health degrees in 2020, 265 of 392 institutions remain (data not shown). It is not clear whether the differences represent true, small programs or reporting errors; these affect institution totals but do not materially affect conferral totals (these institutions represented 3.1% of conferrals in 2020).

Second, UGPHD majors are reported; public health minors are not included, thus excluding from our analysis a potentially important indicator of interest in and exposure to public health at the undergraduate level. Third, ASPPH member programs that report graduate outcomes use myriad approaches in data collection. Some augment with administrative data or publicly available data (e.g., LinkedIn scraping). As such, especially in early years of reporting, there are relatively high proportions of unknown employment sectors for employed graduates.

Lastly, a final set of limitations relate to College Scorecard debt data. NCES censors institutions when there are too few records either on salaries or on debt to ensure confidentiality of responses. As such, some institutions are not represented in this data set. Debt data include Parent Plus loans and federal direct subsidized and unsubsidized loans (Stafford loans), but do not include Perkins loans.[33] As such, data may be limited with respect to parental loan reporting around private-backed loans, which are again becoming more common in recent years.

Conclusions

Throughout the past 2 decades, there have been calls for undergraduate public health education to create a greater population-based understanding for, and higher value of, the field of public health.[6,17,34] Thoughtfully developed undergraduate programs have provided, and will continue to provide, a public health foundation to all professions, regardless of the graduate's immediate employment sector. Our data show undergraduate public health graduates have most often entered either the health care or for-profit sectors, and relatively less into governmental public health. The nation relies on the vital roles that governmental public health agencies provide, but a post–COVID-19 world, one with a depleted governmental public health workforce,[18,35] presents grand challenges to protecting the public's health. However, our data show that the nation also has more than 18 000 undergraduate public health graduates each year, which highlights the potential role of undergraduate education in addressing the near-future governmental public health gaps as well as an opportunity to recruit a more diverse and representative workforce. AJPH

ABOUT THE AUTHORS

Jonathon P. Leider and Chelsey Kirkland are with the Center for Public Health Systems in the Division of Health Policy and Management, University of Minnesota School of Public Health, Minneapolis. Emily Burke, Christine Plepys, and Laura Magaña are with the Association of Schools and Programs of Public Health, Washington, DC. Ruby H. N. Nguyen is with the Division of Epidemiology and Community Health, University of Minnesota School of Public Health. Beth Resnick is with the Johns

Hopkins Bloomberg School of Public Health, Department of Health Policy and Management, Baltimore, MD.

CORRESPONDENCE

Correspondence should be sent to Jonathon Leider, D312 Mayo Building, MMC 729, 420 Delaware St SE, Minneapolis, MN 55455 (e-mail: leider@umn.edu). Reprints can be ordered at https://ajph.org by clicking the "Reprints" link.

PUBLICATION INFORMATION

Full Citation: Leider JP, Burke E, Nguyen RHN, et al. Trends in degree conferrals, degree-associated debt, and employment outcomes among undergraduate public health degree graduates, 2001–2020. *Am J Public Health*. 2023;113(1): 115–123.

Acceptance Date: August 29, 2022.

DOI: https://doi.org/10.2105/AJPH.2022.307113

CONTRIBUTORS

J. P. Leider, E. Burke, and C. Kirkland conducted initial analyses. All authors drafted the initial document and provided edits and critical review.

CONFLICTS OF INTEREST

The authors have no items to disclose.

HUMAN PARTICIPANT PROTECTION

The project involved secondary data analysis of publicly available data and employment outcomes data for Association of Schools and Programs of Public Health alumni institutions.

REFERENCES

1. Leider JP, Resnick B, Erwin P. Educated citizenry or workforce pipeline development? Questions for the future of undergraduate public health in the United States. *Am J Public Health*. 2022;112(4): 582–585. https://doi.org/10.2105/AJPH.2022.306742
2. Rosenfield A, Morse SS, Yanda K. September 11: the response and role of public health. *Am J Public Health*. 2002;92(1):10–11. https://doi.org/10.2105/AJPH.92.1.10
3. Institute of Medicine. *The Future of the Public's Health in the 21st Century*. Washington, DC: National Academy Press; 2003.
4. Riegelman RK, Albertine S, Wykoff R. A history of undergraduate education for public health: from behind the scenes to center stage. *Front Public Health*. 2015;3:70. https://doi.org/10.3389/fpubh.2015.00070
5. Leider JP, Castrucci BC, Plepys CM, Blakely C, Burke E, Sprague JB. On academics: characterizing the growth of the undergraduate public health major: US, 1992–2012. *Public Health Rep*. 2015;130(1):104–113. https://doi.org/10.1177/003335491513000114
6. Resnick B, Leider JP, Riegelman R. The landscape of US undergraduate public health education. *Public Health Rep*. 2018;133(5):619–628. https://doi.org/10.1177/0033354918784911
7. Council on Education for Public Health. Council on Education for Public Health history. 2015. Available at: https://ceph.org/about/org-info. Accessed October 20, 2022.
8. Council on Education for Public Health. List of accredited schools and programs. Available at: https://ceph.org/about/org-info/who-we-accredit/accredited. Accessed March 13, 2022.
9. Erwin PC, Beck AJ, Yeager VA, Leider JP. Public health undergraduates in the workforce: a trickle, soon a wave? *Am J Public Health*. 2019;109(5): 685–687. https://doi.org/10.2105/AJPH.2019.305004
10. Lee JM, Kleinbaum D, Diener-West M, et al. Teaching excellence in public health: a call to action. *Public Health Rep*. 2008;123(3):405–407. https://doi.org/10.1177/003335490812300324
11. Matsusaki T, Sakai T. The role of certified registered nurse anesthetists in the United States. *J Anesth*. 2011;25(5):734–740. https://doi.org/10.1007/s00540-011-1193-5
12. Hoyem RL, Quraishi JA, Jordan L, Wiltse Nicely KL. Advocacy, research, and anesthesia practice models: key studies of safety and cost-effectiveness. *Policy Polit Nurs Pract*. 2019;20(4):193–204. https://doi.org/10.1177/1527154419874410
13. National Center for Education Statistics. Integrated Postsecondary Education Data System. 2020. Available at: https://nces.ed.gov/ipeds/use-the-data. Accessed October 20, 2022.
14. Association of Schools and Programs of Public Health. About. Available at: https://aspph.org/about. Accessed March 13, 2022.
15. Council on Education for Public Health. Date of initial accreditation (retroactive accreditation). Available at: https://ceph.org/constituents/schools/faqs/general/date-of-initial-accreditation-retroactive-accreditation. Accessed March 13, 2022.
16. Plepys CM, Krasna H, Leider JP, Burke EM, Blakely CH, Magana L. First-destination outcomes for 2015–2018 public health graduates: focus on employment. *Am J Public Health*. 2021;111(3): 475–484. https://doi.org/10.2105/AJPH.2020.306038
17. Lee JM. Articulation of undergraduate and graduate education in public health. *Public Health Rep*. 2008;123(suppl 2):12–17. https://doi.org/10.1177/00333549081230S203
18. de Beaumont Foundation, PHNCI. Staffing up: workforce levels needed to provide basic public health services for all Americans. October 2021. Available at: https://phnci.org/uploads/resource-files/Staffing-Up-Research-Brief.pdf. Accessed October 20, 2022.
19. Hall K, Brees K, McCall TC, Cunningham MC, Alford AA. Forces of change: the COVID-19 edition. National Association of County and City Health Officials. 2022. Available at: https://www.naccho.org/uploads/downloadable-resources/2020-Forces-of-Change-The-COVID-19-Edition.pdf. Accessed October 20, 2022.
20. The 2021 Public Health Workforce Interests and Needs Survey. Bethesda, MD: de Beaumont Foundation; 2022.
21. Horney JA, Davis M, Ricchetti-Masterson KL, Macdonald PDM. Fueling the public health workforce pipeline through student surge capacity response teams. *J Community Health*. 2014;39(1):35–39. https://doi.org/10.1007/s10900-013-9750-5
22. McClamroch KJ, Montgomery JP. Epidemiology for high school students: improving the public health pipeline. *Public Health Rep*. 2009;124(6): 898–904. https://doi.org/10.1177/003335490912400620
23. Yeager VA, Beitsch LM, Hasbrouck L. A mismatch between the educational pipeline and public health workforce: can it be reconciled? *Public Health Rep*. 2016;131(3):507–509. https://doi.org/10.1177/003335491613100318
24. Krasna H, Fried L. Generation public health: fixing the broken bridge between public health education and the governmental workforce. *Am J Public Health*. 2021;111(8):1413–1417. https://doi.org/10.2105/AJPH.2021.306317
25. Locke R, McGinty M, Guerrero Ramirez G, Sellers K. Attracting new talent to the governmental public health workforce: strategies for improved recruitment of public health graduates. *J Public Health Manag Pract*. 2022;28(1):E235–E243. https://doi.org/10.1097/PHH.0000000000001336
26. National Center for Education Statistics. Total fall enrollment in degree-granting postsecondary institutions, by attendance status, sex, and age of student: selected years, 2001 through 2030. Washington, DC: US Department of Education, Integrated Postsecondary Education Data System; 2022.
27. National Student Clearinghouse Research Center. National college progression rates. 2021. Available at: https://nscresearchcenter.org/wp-content/uploads/2021_HSBenchmarksCovidReport.pdf. Accessed October 20, 2022.
28. Krupnick M. More students are dropping out of college during Covid—and it could get worse. 2022. Available at: https://hechingerreport.org/more-students-are-dropping-out-of-college-during-covid-and-it-could-get-worse. Accessed April 14, 2022.
29. Foote A, Grosz M. The effect of local labor market downturns on postsecondary enrollment and program choice. *Educ Finance Policy*. 2020;15(4): 593–622. https://doi.org/10.1162/edfp_a_00288
30. Lederman D. Online is (increasingly) local. 2019. Available at: https://www.insidehighered.com/digital-learning/article/2019/06/05/annual-survey-shows-online-college-students-increasingly. Accessed April 14, 2022.
31. Nakae S, Porfeli EJ, Davis D, et al. Enrollment management in undergraduate medical school admissions: a complementary framework to holistic review for increasing diversity in medicine. *Acad Med*. 2021;96(4):501–506. https://doi.org/10.1097/ACM.0000000000003866
32. Leider JP, Plepys CM, Castrucci BC, Burke EM, Blakely CH. Trends in the conferral of graduate public health degrees: a triangulated approach. *Public Health Rep*. 2018;133(6):729–737. https://doi.org/10.1177/0033354918791542
33. Technical documentation: college scorecard data by field of study. Washington, DC: National Center for Education Statistics; 2022.
34. Petersen DJ, Albertine S, Plepys CM, Calhoun JG. Developing an educated citizenry: the undergraduate public health learning outcomes project. *Public Health Rep*. 2013;128(5):425–430. https://doi.org/10.1177/003335491312800517
35. Krasna H, Kornfeld J, Cushman L, Ni S, Antoniou P, March D. The new public health workforce: employment outcomes of public health graduate students. *J Public Health Manag Pract*. 2021;27(1): 12–19. https://doi.org/10.1097/PHH.0000000000000976

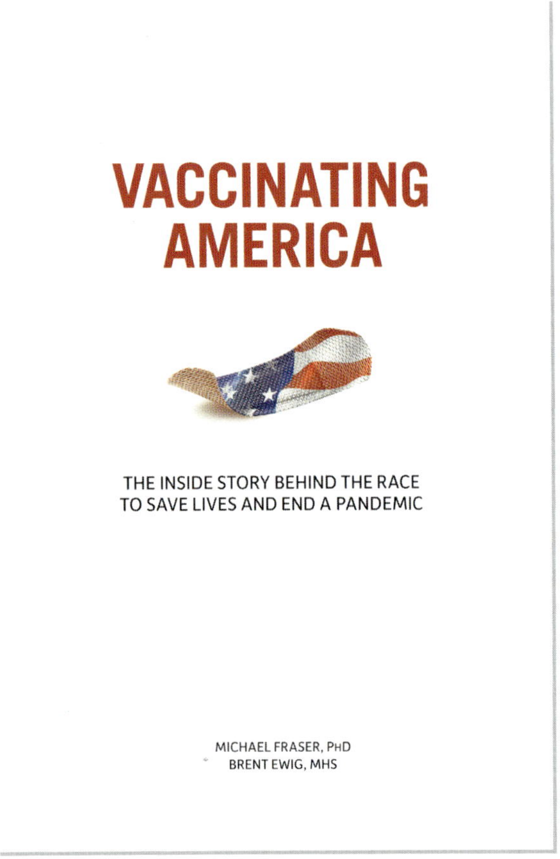

Vaccinating America: The Inside Story Behind the Race to Save Lives, and End a Pandemic

Edited by: Michael Fraser, PhD, Brent Ewig, MHS

2023, 250 PP, SFTCVR, ISBN 978-0-87553-332-2

Vaccinating America spotlights the public servants and heroes who planned and executed this unprecedented program to combat COVID-19 amidst fierce partisan divides, bureaucratic infighting and overwhelming logistical challenges, and doesn't hold back on pointing out those who hindered progress.

APHABOOKSTORE.ORG

APHA PRESS

AN IMPRINT OF AMERICAN PUBLIC HEALTH ASSOCIATION